Cannabi

An Introduction to Cannabis for Consumers, Producers, Providers, Policy Makers, and Health Professionals

Collaboratively written by:
Joshua T. Winningham, Pharm.D,
Abigail M. Testaberg, Jesse Long and
Buck Duncan on behalf of
PhytoPharm.D, LLC and
Whole Plant Technologies, Inc.

Content editor:
Jody Testaberg

Copy editor:
Shelbey Winningham

Administrative contributions by:
Emily DeYmaz and Collin Paschke

Cover design and layout by:
Jeff Reisdorfer

Cannabis Primer: An Introduction to Cannabis for Consumers, Producers, Providers, Policy Makers, and Health Professionals

Copyright © 2019 by PhytoPharm.D, LLC

Dedication

Renee Tomal and William Matthew Lynch

Disclaimer

The possession, distribution, and manufacturing of cannabis and cannabis-based products (specifically defined as "marihuana" under Title 21 United States Code (USC) Controlled Substances Act Section 802) are illegal under federal law. Federal law currently conflicts with laws in some states. Some state laws may, in some jurisdictions, decriminalize such activity under certain circumstances, but compliance with state law does not confer immunity from federal enforcement policies.

The United States Drug Enforcement Administration does not recognize cannabis to have any medical value. This book is not intended as a substitute for professional medical advice, diagnosis, or treatment. All content published here within is for educational purposes only. Always seek the advice of your physician or other qualified health provider with any questions you may have regarding a medical condition. Never disregard professional medical advice or delay in seeking it because of something you have read in this book. If you think you may have a medical emergency, call your doctor, go to the emergency department, or call 911 immediately.

The authors of this book have published, to the best of their abilities, the most current information. However, there may be mistakes in the text that the authors were unable to detect. The information presented is not exhaustive and does not cover all aspects of cannabis. Materials published here within are for the purpose of education on cannabis topics and the information should not be considered complete, nor should it be relied on to suggest a definitive course of treatment for a particular individual. It should not be used in place of a visit, call, consultation, or the advice of your physician or other qualified healthcare providers.

This book does not offer any specific recommendations for individual cannabis products. Cannabis products cannot be approved by the FDA, therefore cannot make authorized health, structure or function claims. Unqualified health claims describing the effect a substance has on reducing the risk of, or preventing, a disease must follow submission guidelines in the FDA Code of Federal Regulations Title 21 - including the disclaimer: "These statements have not been evaluated by the Food and Drug Administration. This product is not intended to diagnose, treat, cure, or prevent any disease." Always consult with your physician or other qualified healthcare provider before consuming cannabis.

Table of Contents

Opening Note

While there are many terms for cannabis and language is fluid, there are negative connotations with the term marijuana (which we will explore) that continue to be wielded for political gain. Since cannabis is the accepted botanical term for the genus, and carries less historiographical weight, the cannabis community has made strides to eliminate marijuana from the medical vernacular. Following suit, we will use the term cannabis throughout this book. Any other term used for cannabis (marihuana, marijuana...) will be used only in given titles of an organized group or when quoting a cited source.

Section 1:
History of Cannabis

Chapter 1: Origins

Anatomically modern humans (Homo sapiens) evolved nearly a quarter million years ago. There is currently no evidence that humans used agricultural methods prior to 15,000-20,000 years ago. Theories conjecture a warming climate and/or intellectual advances led to the invention of agriculture; stone tools were modified to help sow plants into the softening earth.[1] The period of climate warming, agriculture invention, and new stone tools is called the Neolithic Age (New Stone Age).

Ancestors of the cannabis plant evolved over 100,000 years ago in Central Eurasia.[2] Prior to the Neolithic Revolution (also known as the Agricultural Revolution), there is no evidence of how hunter-gatherers interfaced with the cannabis plant, though cannabis seeds would have been a source of nutrition. It is also thought that hunter-gatherers used various drug-plants for medicine, including spiritual experiences, as early as the Paleolithic Era (Old Stone age).[3] The earliest archaeological evidence of cannabis as an agricultural crop comes from the steppe regions of Central Asia, or China, approximately 5-6,000 years ago. Various regional groups used the cannabis plant for a variety of different purposes including food, oil, fiber, and medicine (including an intoxicant associated with ritual).[4]

From Central Eurasia, cannabis was spread outside of the region by both natural phenomena and humans. Consequently, cannabis grew as both a wild and cultivated plant in regions across the world. Cannabis plants that developed a consistent set of characteristics through adaptation and/or cultivation are referred to as landrace strains. Over the past 10,000 years, landrace strains used for food, oil, fiber, and/or medicine developed all around the world as a cash crop and a driver of trade.

Chinese written text from the first century AD gestures to the use of cannabis as medicine as early as 2,900 BC for such conditions as gout, rheumatism, and malaria. In the second century AD, cannabis combined with alcohol was used as an anesthetic in China. An Indian book written between 2000 and 1400 BC discusses the anti-anxiety properties of cannabis, which was often consumed as a milk-tea with other herbs and referred to as bhang. Medical application, such as fever reducer, digestive regulator, and mood elevator, of bhang is cited by the Indian government into the late 1800s. A first century AD Greek collection on medicinal herbs discussed cannabis as a remedy for earaches and such was documented into the 1500s.[5]

Chapter 2: Cannabis in Early America

Cannabis was introduced to North and South America in the 1500s.[6] The Spanish first cultivated cannabis in their colonies in the sixteenth century. The French and British began cultivation in the early 1600s, including plantings in Port Royal, Virginia, and Plymouth. The European colonizers primarily produced cannabis for fiber (mainly for shipping rope) rather than for an intoxicant or medicine. In the southern hemisphere, Brazil for example, slaves brought with them the tradition of using cannabis for medical and social purposes. This practice was adopted by some of the indigenous groups as well. French and British slaves did not seem to carry as many traditions with cannabis, presumably because they were enslaved from different regions in Africa with different cultural practices.[7] There is evidence, however, that North American cannabis farmers did smoke their crop in addition to using it for industrial purposes. Presidents Washington and Jefferson were cannabis farmers, and letters and diaries support that they smoked their crop as an alternative to tobacco and alcohol.[8]
[9] [10]

Despite historically and geographically widespread use of cannabis as medicine or ritual in China, the Middle (and Near) East, Africa, and South America, there was limited medical/ritual usage of cannabis in Europe and North America until the turn of the nineteenth century. French psychiatrist Jacques-Joseph Moreau and Irish physician William B. O'Shaughnessy introduced medical use of cannabis into Western medicine in the mid 1800s:

> Cannabis drug preparations were extensively used in the West between the middle of the nineteenth century and World War II, particularly as a substitute for opiates, and as antispasmodic, analgesic, hypnotic, and sedative agents (Mikuriya 1969). Cannabis was used to treat a very wide range of ailments, including insomnia, headaches, anorexia, sexual dysfunction, whooping cough and asthma.

Orally administered tinctures, especially alcoholic, were particularly popular, with hundreds of brands in circulation (Frankhauser 2002).[11]

In the United States, cannabis was commonly used as medicine and was available for purchase in pharmacies, and general stores, from the mid 1800s until 1915.

Chapter 3: Prohibition of Intoxicants

Until the Mexican Revolution in 1910, United States production and consumption of cannabis was predominantly for industrial fiber or pharmaceutical purposes. Spiritual, ritual, social, and/ or recreational use of cannabis still remained uncommon in North America. The unrest of the Mexican Revolution resulted in large immigrant populations settling in the Southwestern United States. Mexican immigrants brought with them the traditions of social use of cannabis, which had been passed to them via Central African slaves brought to South America:

> Historically, the earliest and most numerous group of users in the Americas were slaves from western Central Africa (modern Gabon to Angola). Their words for cannabis are now used in nearly all the places they (involuntarily) ended up during the 1700s and 1800s, which includes West Africa, the Caribbean and South America. Most notably, in Central America, the Kimbundu (Angolan) word mariamba became the Spanish word marihuana.[12]

Racism and anti-immigration sentiment resulted in border states strategizing to exert power and control over the immigrants. One of many tactics used was to isolate association of cannabis with the immigrant population, popularize the word marihuana instead of cannabis, and then vilify "marihuana" consumption as dangerous and as a societal threat.[13] Many individual states passed laws against various intoxicants throughout the early 1900s.

Cannabis vilification, vis-á-vis Mexican immigration, coincided with a larger Federal push to regulate pharmaceuticals and psychoactive substances. The 1906 United States *Pure Food and Drug Act* called for appropriate labeling of the quantity or proportion of any alcohol, morphine, opium, cocaine, heroin, alpha or beta eucaine, chloroform, cannabis indica, chloral hydrate, or acetanilide within foods and drugs. The 1909 *Opium Exclusion Act* banned the importation of smoking opium, thereby creating the first illegal drug. The 1914 *Harrison Narcotics Act* regulated opiates (including morphine and heroin) from being grown or distributed and required a physician prescription for use. Despite cocaine not being an opiate, it was also included in the *Harrison Narcotic Act*. In 1919, the *Volstead Act* made the 18th amendment to the Constitution, which banned the sale, production, and transportation of alcohol. Alcohol prohibition was repealed in 1933 under the ratification of the 21st amendment to the Constitution. The 1924 *Anti-Heroin Act* prohibited the importation and production of opium into heroin. In 1937, the *Marijuana Tax Act* criminalized the possession of cannabis by restricting possession and production to those who paid an excise tax for certain authorized medical and industrial uses, but there was no application process initiated to receive the authorized stamp, so cannabis production and possession was essentially outlawed.[14]

In 1970, the *Comprehensive Drug Abuse Prevention and Control Act* (CDAPC) was enacted. It was designed to organize the array of Federal drug laws that preceded it into an ordered system. The act had three parts including a substance abuse program, production/distribution/possession regulation, and import/export laws. The second part, regarding regulation of controlled substances (*Controlled Substances Act* [CSA]), created five categories (schedules) of drugs and sorted individual drugs into the schedules based on a list of criteria describing each drug's potential danger, propensity for abuse, and possible medical use with Schedule I drugs being the most dangerous, addictive, and least medicinal. Cannabis, referred to as marihuana, was placed as a Schedule I drug, where it remains today.

Chapter 4: Factors Contributing to Prohibition

A variety of factors in the twentieth century lead to the prohibition of intoxicants. Technological, racial, political, economic, and philosophical factors all contributed to the prohibition of intoxicants.

Technology

Nineteenth century advancements in biochemistry, biotechnology, pharmacy, and marketing introduced larger distribution of more potent intoxicants into cultural use:

> Until the 19th century, drugs had been used for millennia in their natural form. Cocaine and morphine, for example, were available only in coca leaves or poppy plants that were chewed, dissolved in alcoholic beverages or taken in some way that diluted the impact of the active agent. The advent of organic chemistry in the 1800s changed the available forms of these drugs. Morphine was isolated in the first decade and cocaine by 1860; In 1874 diacetylmorphine was synthesized from morphine (although it became better known as heroin when the Bayer Company introduced it in 1898). By mid-century the hypodermic syringe was perfected, and by 1870 it had become a familiar instrument to American physicians and patients [...] At the same time, the astounding growth of the pharmaceutical industry intensified the ramifications of these accomplishments. As the century wore on, manufacturers grew increasingly adept at exploiting a marketable innovation and moving it into mass production, as well as advertising and distributing it throughout the world.[15]

Concentrated, readily available, and highly marketed opium (and derivatives morphine and heroin) and cocaine became less benign than intoxicants like sugar, tea, and coffee, and were causing increased addiction ills and societal disruptions.

Prohibitionist culture grouped cannabis and alcohol with opium and cocaine. Much later, it added other hallucinogens, such as mescaline and lysergic acid diethylamide (LSD). Even in concentrated form, hallucinogens (including cannabis) do not have the same toxic and lethal nature as alcohol, opium, and cocaine.

Race and Politics

In many instances, white patriarchy demonized social drugs of choice of whichever racial group it wanted to exert power and control over. Early 1900s regulation of smokable opium targeted Chinese immigrants in San Francisco. Early-to-mid 1900s prohibition of cannabis targeted Mexican immigrants and the Harlem Renaissance. 1970s tightening of prohibition regulations targeted Southern Black voters.[16]

Similar tactics used against specific racial groups were also used against broader political foes. In the 1960s, a strong counterculture movement arose against government overreach at home and abroad. Young adults and minorities questioned lack of civil rights and liberties, effects of corporate greed (and government corruption) on the environment and health and wellbeing of the citizenry, and wars being fought abroad that seemed to be about capitalist enterprise rather than self-defense or social justice. Civil Rights groups, United Farm Workers, Hippies, Anti-war Protesters, Environmentalists, and others, were grouped into one "counterculture." Many counter culturalists questioned, and defied, drug prohibition as well. Despite early twentieth century drug prohibition, interest in, research around, and use of illicit drugs emerged and became visible to society beyond the shadows. Vilification of these groups through their illicit drug use helped delegitimize their political power. Tightening of prohibition regulation allowed a mechanism for control.[17]

Economics

Industrial Capitalism

The second phase of the Industrial Revolution from the late 1800s to the early 1900s resulted in rapid urbanization, mass immigration, overcrowded cities, health and safety concerns, and exploitative working conditions that resulted in a large population of poor, uneducated, and economically immobile citizens. Prohibition rhetoric blamed negative societal conditions on intoxicants instead of focusing attention on (and solving) the negative aspects of the capitalist driven Industrial Revolution—notably corporate greed and government corruption.[18]

Capitalist Trade

In the late 1700s, England conquered India and Burma. In order to pay for the colonization of India and Burma, England needed a new revenue source. They found it in the taxes on British merchants shipping opium to China. Historically, China's opium market was similar to the alcohol and tobacco market in the West; opium was treated as a cash crop for socially approved consumption. British merchant flooding of China's opium market, as well as British competition with China's own export market, resulted in China shutting down opium importation. British merchants continued to import opium illegally. Two wars were fought between China and England, in-part over the import/export of opium. The decentralized nature of the early United States (more state control with little Federal oversight) did not initially allow the United States to combat opium entering the country. As the Federal government implemented prohibition, they were also able to implement trade controls in an attempt to reduce intoxicants entering the country.[19]

Interest Groups

"Rent seeking" is the quest for privileged benefits from a government for economic gain of a group, or individual, without benefiting the society through broader wealth creation.[20]

23

Rent-seeking can be done in many ways, including: running for office with personal or group interests in mind, donations to a political candidate or party to influence decision making, influencing voter turnout, or lobbying (influencing the government to act in a way beneficial to a person, or group).

Intoxicant prohibition had many rent seekers. The American Medical Association (AMA), American Pharmaceutical Association, The National Drug Wholesalers Association, and the Association of the Retail Druggists all came into being in the mid-to-late 1800s. Today physicians diagnose patients, pharmacists dispense drugs, and pharmaceutical companies make drugs, but when these industries were first emerging, the roles were convoluted and lacked professional standards. As the Western medical industry took shape, a common factor all associations strategized around was controlling drugs.[21]

Other rent seekers, prompting cannabis-specific prohibition in 1937 via the *Marijuana Tax Act,* are less obvious. Primary source evidence of the "Corporate Conspiracy" against hemp in the 1930s is lacking. However, general rent seeking behaviors of the DuPont Corporation in that era are well documented.[22] DuPont Corporation had petroleum synthetic fiber (nylon) technology, wood-pulp paper technology, and a variety of chemical technologies (pesticides, herbicides, and fertilizers) used extensively by the cotton industry. DuPont's obvious general rent seeking behaviors, as well as technologies with which cannabis directly competed, has fueled long standing belief that they played a role in cannabis prohibition.

It is also widely argued that a government agency itself (via Harry Anslinger and the Federal Narcotics Bureau [FNB]) was a rent seeker in cannabis prohibition.[23] Three years prior to the failing of alcohol prohibition, Anslinger was reassigned to the Narcotics Division to clean up mob-related corruption in the narcotics arm of the Prohibition Unit. The government also moved the Narcotics Unit out of the Prohibition Unit and (through the *Porter Act* of 1930) created a new arm of the Treasury Department: the FNB. By 1935, the new agency was already at risk due to budget concerns stemming

24

from The Great Depression. In addition, Anslinger struggled to keep state agencies in-line with the FNB. Out of these circumstances, a push for cannabis prohibition was not invented by Anslinger, but rather used as a rent seeking tactic:

> Contrary to pop history, Harry Anslinger did not start America's legendary campaign against marijuana. In fact he tried to keep the Bureau out of cannabis enforcement in the beginning because he thought eradication would be impossible. The stuff grows, he said, "like dandelions."(24) But after the curtain came down on Prohibition, the nation's moral focus moved on to the next available villain, and the marijuana issue was waiting in the wings. By 1933 several states had already outlawed the Devil Weed and some officials were calling for a national ban. Anslinger realized he might be able to use this issue as a weapon - a club to whip the states into line. He needed to get local law enforcement more involved in the battle against narcotics because his tiny force of 250 agents could barely keep track of the major traffickers.(25) For months Anslinger had been on the road trying to convince the states to adopt some kind of uniform narcotics enforcement, and he was getting nowhere. The state governments were as strapped as Washington. So sometime in 1935 he decided to build a little fire and he suddenly upgraded marijuana from a low priority nuisance to an "evil as hellish as heroin."(26)[24]

Cannabis fear-mongering was a tactic used by Anslinger to breath necessity into the Federal agency he was employed.

Philosophy

Social and political philosophies of the late nineteenth and early twentieth centuries also played a significant role in prohibition culture. The Temperance Movement, which criticized alcohol intoxication and promoted abstinence, began in the early nineteenth century. Millennial shifts in both the nineteenth and twentieth centuries saw surges in Christian fundamentalism. Religious fervor in preparation of the second coming of Christ often included abstinence from alcohol on the path to salvation. Toward the end of the 1800s, leadership from all facets of society (church, politics, business, and social reform) showed increasing concern over alcohol consumption in the United States. However, with a history of fundamentalism, evangelical Protestants became more vigilant and vocal regarding alcohol prohibition.[25]

Another movement that influenced prohibition was rooted in a spirit of reform that swept the United States at the beginning of the twentieth century. Big Business was rapidly changing the United States landscape. Rural farmers were being affected by overproduction and unfair pricing by monopolistic railroads and grain elevators.[26] The Industrial Revolution caused migration from rural areas, mass immigration, and rapid urbanization. The rich and middle class experienced positive outcomes from industrialization including advances in transportation that allowed them to live outside the inner city. The working class poor living in the city experienced overcrowding, poor infrastructure, pollution, and terrible working conditions including: mass immigration, long working hours, low wages, and unsafe working conditions (such as child labor). These issues coalesced into increased crime and disease.

The Progressive Era was a response to the negative impacts of Big Business and Industrialization. Rather than argue against Modernization, Progressives believed they could create a balance of equitable standards of living and promotion of human advancement through laws and institutions:

> Whether the particular task into which they plunged was raising the quality of life for the urban working class, conserving natural resources, establishing professional societies and standards, improving governmental morality, democracy, and services, or controlling business practices, progressives repeatedly displayed their unshakable confidence that legal and bureaucratic instruments could be found which would permanently uplift that aspect of their environment.[27]

Intoxicant prohibition fit into Progressive Era philosophy. Instead of seeing the capitalist construct at odds with fostering a positive human condition, in their perception, alcohol and drugs affected a person's ability to perform their job and caused problems in society. Progressives pushed for social reform, regulation, and prohibition for the good of their perceived notions of societal progress.

Another movement that propelled prohibition culture was increased Patriotism and the rise of the National spirit that came during World War I. With little questioning, United States citizens were willing to give up individual freedoms for the good of the country. In addition, the war centralized authority at the Federal level and allowed the Federal government more control over economic aspects of the country for the war effort.[28]

Chapter 5: Unintended Consequences of Prohibition and The War on Drugs

The alcohol prohibition experience in the United States made clear unintended consequences of intoxicant prohibition in general. Alcohol prohibition increased criminal activity, increased government corruption, increased the need for funding for enforcement, increased prosecutions (which held up the courts), increased court involvement in oversight of Federal agencies (which undermined the power of the state over individual liberties), decreased tax revenue, crippled ancillary industries, and demonized persons with addiction issues, leaving them fewer social supports for help.[29] Many of these factors contributed to the failure of alcohol prohibition, but the two factors most widely credited with the repeal of the 18th Amendment are the wide use (and acceptance) of alcohol before (and during) prohibition, and inadequate organization (and funding) to enforce prohibition.

Learning from the failures of alcohol prohibition, the *CDAPC Act* of 1970 took into consideration the need to enforce the regulatory and prohibitionist laws. The Drug Enforcement Agency (DEA), supervised by the United States Attorney General (USAG), was created three years after the *CSA* in order to enforce the Act. A much smaller consumption population, improved system for enforcement, and a calculated "War on Drugs" government marketing campaign (coined by President Nixon, but amplified by subsequent political agents to this day) provided a framework for drug prohibition to succeed when alcohol prohibition had not.

United States drug policy significantly influenced international drug policy. For over a century (since opium prohibition and the Shanghai Commission) the United States has attempted to blame international players for domestic drug use and has used trade agreements and international relations to influence global drug prohibition.

The birth of the United Nations and eventual creation of the United Nations Commission on Narcotic Drugs—a commision of the United Nations Economic and Social Council and central drug-policy making body—extended the United States authority on the War on Drugs.[30]

Domestic Consequences

Copious government spending, rise in organized crime, increased corruption by government agencies, flooding of the criminal court system, mass incarceration, creation of the private prison system, and infringement on civil liberties are all consequences the Drug War has had on the United States Justice system:

> Drug policy has become a major force in the lives of millions of persons caught in the justice system; the same holds true for millions of their family members, relatives, and friends; and the inner-city communities that suffer as a result of the policies emanating from this state-constructed moral panic.[31]

The majority of people arrested, prosecuted, and jailed for drugs are non-violent, low-level offenders. These shifts in the Justice system have disproportionately affected people of color and the poor, which has influenced a variety of social concerns. While not exhaustive, these concerns include unemployment, decline in marriage, urban violence, increased risk in the spread of HIV (via exposure through incarceration), and voting disenfranchisement.

Global Consequences

Despite nearly forty years of fighting the Drug War, the United Nations Office on Drug and Crime estimated in 2009 between 155 and 250 million people globally, or 3.5% to 5.7% of the population aged 15-64, had used illicit substances at least once. Cannabis users constitute 129-190 million of those people, while amphetamine-type stimulants make up the second most commonly used illicit drug, followed by opiates and cocaine. Opiates were ranked at the top in terms of harm associated.[32] From 1998 to 2008 opiate use increased 34.5%, cocaine use increased 27%, and cannabis use increased 8.5%:

> While accurate estimates of global consumption across the entire 50-year period are not available, an analysis of the last 10 years alone shows a large and growing market.[33]

The United States statistics as of 2013 show similar trends, but with an overall higher percentage of the total population (9%) having had used an illicit drug in the previous month.[34]

Global consequences of the failed War on Drugs, in many ways, mirror outcomes in the United States. Dangerous drug cartels exist all over the world. Cartels bribe corrupt governments from local to state-level authorities. Money made from trafficking is invested in advances in criminal enterprising. Cartels often cooperate with (and fund) radical political organizations and/or agents of other organized crime, such as human trafficking, cyber warfare, counterfeiting, and/ or terrorism. Simply stated, cartel-culture equates to a significant drug trafficking death toll.[35]

In addition to bolstering, rather than eliminating, the production and distribution of illicit drugs, the Drug War has had lasting consequences on global consumers. Resources funnelled to regulation and prohibition of drugs take away from resources needed to help individuals suffering from actual addiction. International public policy and trade agreements linked to The War on Drugs impinge needed resources for other health and human service programs including disease prevention. The Drug War has also demonized and criminalized populations of people for some consumption behaviors that have historically been culturally acceptable and benign.[36]

Chapter 6: Legalization Momentum

Decriminalization

There was pushback against the CSA regarding the medical use of cannabis almost immediately. Oregon decriminalized cannabis in 1973. Since then a dozen states have decriminalized cannabis to some degree. Decriminalization changed cannabis possession from a criminal to a civil offense punishable by fines instead of jail. Each state's decriminalization laws are different with ranging civil penalties and safety from jail sentences.[37]

Research Programs

In 1975 Robert Randall, who was growing his own cannabis to self-treat glaucoma, was arrested for possession. Randall fought the charges in court using a "medical necessity" defense, and he won. As a result, Randall became the first patient to receive medical cannabis from the government under the Investigational New Drug program which allowed patients to receive non-FDA approved drugs on an investigational basis.

The program was very small for a long time, but in 1992 a slew of patients applied for the program. The increased interest in the program was partly a result of common knowledge that cannabis helped HIV/AIDS patients with wasting syndrome and nausea. As the program was receiving new interest, President Bush shut down the program.

Using some of the same principles of the *Investigational New Drug Act*, states worked to gain access to cannabis for medical purposes. Lead by New Mexico in 1978, thirty-five states eventually created cannabis research programs in an effort to access Federally produced and distributed cannabis for patients. As the strategy gained popularity, the Federal government began to provide synthetic THC instead of actual cannabis.[38]

33

Rescheduling

In 1981, 1983, and 1985 bills were introduced to move cannabis from schedule I to schedule II, but none gained real traction. From 1984 until 1989, in a series of hearings spurred by a petition submitted to the Federal government in 1972 by the National Organization for the Reform of Marijuana Laws (NORML), the DEA considered the rescheduling of cannabis. In what has become common practice by the DEA, rescheduling was denied in spite of ample evidence for the medical use of cannabis and Agency personnel advisement to reschedule. Amidst this period, a synthetic THC drug, Marinol, was approved by the FDA in 1985.[39]

Initiatives

In the early 1990s, tactics moved away from lobbying the government for access to medical cannabis and toward the initiative process. Ballot initiatives begin with a minimum number of registered voters signing a petition to bring about a public vote on a proposed statute or constitutional amendment. San Francisco and Santa Cruz were the first to successfully pass initiatives that offered localized protection for patients using medical cannabis. In 1996, California passed a statewide initiative that legalized the medical use of cannabis. California's Proposition 215 is also known as the *Compassionate Use Act*.[40] Since California's initiative, seventeen other states have enacted medical cannabis legalization via initiatives.[41]

Bills into Law

Fifteen other states have passed medical cannabis legislation through Congressional bills. Twelve additional states have passed "CBD Only" laws with varied accessibility to patients. Many of the factors that contributed to prohibition in the beginning of the twentieth century continue to play a role in cannabis legalization today.

One of the largest contributing factors of continued cannabis prohibition is latent public sentiment regarding the dangers of cannabis. A century of the perpetuation of myths about cannabis has left much of the citizenry ignorant to what is true and untrue about it. Cannabis is especially interesting because it carries with it both a negative "harmless hippie" reputation as well as an association with more dangerous criminal and disruptive behaviors. Christian evangelical moralists hold steady that cannabis corrupts the soul. Moderate Republicans and Moderate Democrats push for public health policy that keeps the citizenry safe from themselves:

> It would be misleading to suggest that public health researchers inject any kind of traditional Baptist passion into marijuana policy debates; indeed, they try to do just the opposite, emphasizing value-neutral arguments that can be empirically supported. But many of these scholars, who may well be in favor of changing marijuana policies themselves, have nevertheless lent support to the policy status quo by building up the evidentiary record supporting the idea that marijuana is physically and socially harmful, often without giving comparable consideration to the therapeutic or hedonic benefits of responsible marijuana use or to the social costs of the war on drugs.[42]

As we will visit later, cannabis can be addictive, misused, and have negative side effects; however, we are now finding that the negative implications of cannabis consumption pale in comparison to the ethos and are far less problematic than the negative effects of prohibition. National Families in Action, Community Alliances for Drug Free Youth, Parents Opposed to Pot, Citizens Against Legalizing Marijuana, Take Back America Campaign, International Faith Based Coalition, and RAND's Drug Policy Research Center are examples of groups opposing cannabis legalization largely using latent public sentiment of perceived, rather than actual, threats.

Old and new rent seekers also factor into cannabis legalization. Companies involved in mandatory treatment programs lose if the court system cannot offer reduced sentences for voluntary treatment to possession offenders. The alcoholic beverage industry also stands to lose as cannabis is legalized. The beer industry could lose more than $2 billion in retail sales annually due to legal cannabis.[43] Statistics show that beer and liquor sales have declined in states and counties following cannabis legalization:[44] [45]

> ...the California Beer and Beverage Distributors gave $10,000 to the anti-legalization campaign in their state in 2010. But, perhaps because such contributions offer an irresistible target for legalization advocates, alcohol interests have mostly been conspicuous by their absence from the marijuana legalization debate.[46]

Another industry fighting cannabis legalization harkens back to early twentieth century prohibition. As patients replace a variety of pharmaceutical medications with medical cannabis, the pharmaceutical industry could stand to lose $4 billion a year:[47]

> ...many of the researchers who have advocated against legalizing pot have also been on the payroll of leading pharmaceutical firms with products that could be easily replaced by using marijuana. When these individuals have been quoted in the media, their drug-industry ties have not been revealed.[48]

The burgeoning private prison industry stands to lose as cannabis becomes legal. The first private prison corporation, Corrections Corporation of America, was founded in the mid 1980s.[49] A private prison is a privately owned "third party" prison that contracts with the government to detain prisoners. The War on Drugs and Immigration have largely fueled the success of the private prison industry. The growth of private prisons from the 1980s presently is impacted by drug and immigration legislation and shifts in Justice system focus. Harsher sentencing around drugs was enacted in the early 1990s via truth-in-sentencing and three-strikes legislation. This legislation concentrated focus on cannabis possession offenses, seeing 80% of the growth in arrests due to cannabis. Currently, cannabis related offenses account for 45% of yearly arrests. While first-time possession offenses usually do not equate to prison sentences, the legislation for harsher sentences and the "three-strikes" rule began to increase the prison population with low-level cannabis offenders.[50] Corrections Corporation of America (now known as the GEO Group) spends a significant amount of money in lobbying dollars. Some of their lobbying efforts have been associated with anti-legalization efforts.[51] [52]

Government agency rent seeking continues to be a significant force against cannabis legalization:

> Many police officials and prosecutors fear that relaxing marijuana laws will impair their familiar patterns of policing, and many are morally invested in the war on drugs. At the same time, police departments often have their own bootlegger motivation: drug investigations and prosecutions, including those targeting marijuana, are a leading source of asset forfeitures, which provide a significant revenue stream to police and sheriff departments. In Florida, for example, one county sheriff's department's annual strategic plan described marijuana seizures as helping to "meet eligible equipment or other non-recurring needs that could not be met by local funding."25 Enforcement professionals whose expertise (and thus professional standing) revolves around drug enforcement naturally take a special interest in opposing decriminalization. Occasionally, as in the Oregon 2014 election, these forces have managed to contribute six-figure sums to anti-legalization campaigns.[53]

Government institutions, such as the National Institute on Drug Abuse (NIDA) and the White House Office of National Drug Control Policy (ONDCP), have been created to research, develop, and implement social policy perspectives regarding illicit drugs. They exist to mitigate the harms of drug abuse. NIDA currently holds the monopoly (through the University of Mississippi) on cannabis production for research purposes that could lead to FDA approval of cannabis. The ONDCP was responsible for the Drug Abuse

Resistance Education (D.A.R.E.) marketing campaign and education program. These institutions exist on the principle that all illicit drugs are a menace to society. Cannabis legalization erodes this idea and endangers a large portion of what these institutions stand for, as well as their funding.

The DEA has displayed some of the most consistent and strident rent-seeking behaviors through their refusal to acknowledge the safety and medical use of cannabis. If one considers the 1930s Federal Bureau of Narcotics lineage to the DEA, reputable evidence of the general safety and medical value of cannabis has been presented to government narcotics agencies since 1937. During the hearings for the *Marijuana Tax Act*, the AMA argued against the Act, suggesting cannabis be included in the previously enacted *Harrison Narcotics Tax Act* which would have maintained access to cannabis via prescription.[54] Soon after the *Marijuana Tax Act* was passed, New York Mayor Fiorello LaGuardia appointed a commission to research cannabis in New York City, and a report, based on five years of research, was created by the New York Academy of Medicine. Conclusions from the Report include:

> ... 7. The practice of smoking marihuana does not lead to addiction in the medical sense of the word. 8. The sale and distribution of marihuana is not under the control of any single organized group. 9. The use of marihuana does not lead to morphine or heroin or cocaine addiction and no effort is made to create a market for these narcotics by stimulating the practice of marihuana smoking. 10. Marihuana is not the determining factor in the commission of major crimes. 11. Marihuana smoking is not widespread among school children. 12. Juvenile delinquency is not associated with the practice of smoking marihuana. 13. The publicity concerning the catastrophic effects of marihuana smoking in New York City is unfounded.[55]

The report was dismissed by Anslinger and the Federal Bureau of Narcotics as unscientific. In response to the report, Anslinger collaborated with right-wing press and religious groups to defame the report and its creators.[56]

While the CSA was being drafted, Congress mandated a commission to study cannabis. The National Commission on Marihuana and Drug Use (commonly referred to as the Shafer Commission) was created to investigate the facts surrounding cannabis. The placement of cannabis as a schedule I drug preceded the completion of the Commission's report; however, the conclusion of the Commission's report called for the removal of cannabis from Schedule I. Despite President Nixon stacking the Commission to produce, he assumed, an outcome which supported his stance against cannabis,[57] the 1972 report concluded:

> On the basis of our findings, discussed in previous Chapters, we have concluded that society should seek to discourage use, while concentrating its attention on the prevention and treatment of heavy and very heavy use. The Commission feels that the criminalization of possession of marihuana for personal is socially self-defeating as a means of achieving this objective. We have attempted to balance individual freedom on one hand and the obligation of the state to consider the wider social good on the other. We believe our recommended scheme will permit society to exercise its control and influence in ways most useful and efficient, meanwhile reserving to the individual American his sense of privacy, his sense of individuality, and, within the context of all interacting and interdependent society, his options to select his own life style, values, goals and opportunities.[58]

President Nixon ignored the conclusions and recommendations of the report, effectually launched the War on Drugs (including cannabis), and created the DEA as a mechanism to implement oversight and enforcement of the CSA.

In 1988 (in response to the NORML 1972 petition) the DEA requested that Francis Young, an Administrative law judge, consider the merits of rescheduling cannabis from Schedule I to Schedule II. Young concluded:

> The administrative law judge recommends that the Administrator conclude that the marijuana plant considered as a whole has a currently accepted medical use in treatment in the United States, that there is no lack of accepted safety for use of it under medical supervision and that it may lawfully be transferred from Schedule I to Schedule II.[59]

The Administrator of the the DEA, John Lawn, overruled Young's recommendations in 1989, maintaining that cannabis had no medicinal benefit. In 1995, High Times and Jon Gettman (former director of NORML) filed another petition for rescheduling. National Institute of Mental Health studies from 1988 to 1994 on the newly discovered human endocannabinoid system were cited as evidence of the medical value of cannabis.[60] The DEA denied the petition in 2001.[61]

In 2002, Americans for Safe Access and the Coalition for Rescheduling Cannabis filed a petition to consider cannabis for rescheduling. In response, the DEA instructed the United States Department of Health and Human Services to conduct an evaluation of cannabis regarding its scientific and medical merits. The United States Department of Health and Human Services concluded that marijuana has a high potential for abuse, has no accepted medical use in the U.S., and lacks an acceptable level of safety for use even under medical supervision. The DEA Administrator, Michele M. Lionhart, denied the petition in 2011.[62] [63] Both the 2001 and 2011 denials by the DEA were held up in Federal court. Multiple petitions for the rescheduling of cannabis have been denied under the same guidelines of the United States Department of Health and Human Services, rather than new research and/or reports.[64] [65] [66]

40

Adult-use Cannabis

Some states have moved past the question of whether cannabis should be legal for medical use and have also legalized cannabis for adult-use (similar to alcohol and tobacco). Pro-recreational arguments rest on the framework that cannabis is safer than tobacco and alcohol, that sales tax revenue from cannabis can be diverted for government programs, and that an end to prohibition would begin to solve unfair incarceration rates of minorities and the poor. In 2012, Colorado was the first state to legalize adult-use cannabis, which is commonly referred to as recreational cannabis. There are eleven states that allow adult-use cannabis. In January of 2018, Vermont was the first state to do so by passing a law in the legislature rather than via a ballot initiative.

Patchwork Regulation

State-by-state legislation has created different degrees of cannabis legalization and varied regulations for implementation. Some states, like Minnesota, have highly restrictive and regulated markets. Minnesota has two licensed companies to produce and distribute cannabis to patients. There is a limiting list of qualifying conditions that define a patient's ability to access medical cannabis, and smokable flower is not permitted.

New Mexico's medical cannabis program follows a more traditional compassionate care culture similar to the first medical programs initiated up and down the West coast in the late 1990s. Patients still require a qualifying condition diagnosis, but are allowed to grow their own medical cannabis. New Mexico also has a licensing process for non-profit companies to produce and dispense cannabis to patients.

Recreational markets vary in home-grow plant counts (Washington does not allow home-grow), number and size of licensed producers, and testing and tracking regulations.

State vs. Federal Government

No matter state laws, cannabis is still Federally illegal. Generally, the Supremacy Clause of Article VI, cl. 2 of the Constitution of the United States places Federal law at a higher authority over state laws. When a Federal and state law conflict, the state law is usually preempted, or nullified. Court rulings on whether state law conflicts with Federal law regarding cannabis legalization vary. Arguments in favor of Federal preemptive rights of states regarding cannabis are based on the impossibility of a person to participate in a state cannabis program and not be breaking Federal law (impossibility preemption). Also, it is argued that state cannabis laws impede Federal cannabis laws, which also causes conflict (obstacle preemption).[67]

Arguments against Federal preemptive rights are founded on the fact that state laws do not force all citizens to participate in the cannabis programs; therefore, there is a possibility that the laws do not conflict. In addition, there was a precedence that State cannabis legislation was under the authority of State police.[68] In 2005, the Supreme Court case Gonzalez v. Raich argued that the CSA was unconstitutional because it exceeded the Federal government's commerce clause power:

> The district court ruled against the group. The Ninth Circuit Court of Appeals reversed and ruled the CSA unconstitutional as it applied to intrastate (within a state) medical marijuana use. Relying on two U.S. Supreme Court decisions that narrowed Congress' commerce clause power - U.S. v. Lopez (1995) and U.S. v. Morrison (2000) - the Ninth Circuit ruled using medical marijuana did not "substantially affect" interstate commerce and therefore could not be regulated by Congress.[69]

In the final decision:

> ...the Court held that the commerce clause gave Congress authority to prohibit the local cultivation and use of marijuana, despite state law to the contrary. Stevens argued

that the Court's precedent "firmly established" Congress' commerce clause power to regulate purely local activities that are part of a "class of activities" with a substantial effect on interstate commerce. The majority argued that Congress could ban local marijuana use because it was part of such a "class of activities": the national marijuana market. Local use affected supply and demand in the national marijuana market, making the regulation of intrastate use "essential" to regulating the drug's national market.[70]

The 2005 Supreme Court decision spurred increased Federal drug raids in California. Federal (and State) drug raids often result in the collection of (and sometimes the destruction of) cannabis products and the forfeiture of assets related to the trafficking. In many cases, arrests are not made. The DEA has issued a series of memorandums (policies, or guiding principles, not laws) clarifying its stance on medical cannabis programs and addressing its focus for enforcement. The stance these memos take regarding focus of Federal resources against medical cannabis programs have been inconsistent within the same administrations, and even more so as administrative guards change. The 2009 Ogden Memo, which:

> ...provided clear guidance to U.S. attorneys responsible for Federal prosecution under the CSA in the 13 states that had enacted medical cannabis legislation at that time. U.S. attorneys were directed not to prosecute individuals or businesses operating in compliance with state cannabis laws (Ogden, 2009).[71]

...provided an increased sense of security to producers, dispensers, and patients operating within regulatory framework.

The Cole Memos of 2011 and 2013 oscillated between an initial sense of more aggressive Federal enforcement and a significant de-escalation, articulating a Federal hands-off approach to companies and citizens following the laws of the state-regulated cannabis industries.[72] More specifically:

43

...the first Cole memo was interpreted by many as direction for U.S. attorneys to interrogate medical cannabis providers who continued to operate in legal gray areas (Barcott, 2015). Possibly in response to the first Cole memo, medical cannabis patient registrations declined from 2011 to 2013 in Colorado, Montana, and Michigan (Fairman, 2016). However, President Obama stated in November 2012 on national television that cannabis use in states that have passed legalization measures was not a priority for the DOJ (Garvey & Yeh, 2014). A second Cole memo was issued in 2013, after Washington and Colorado had voted to legalize nonmedical cannabis, and more closely reflected President Obama's public statements. This memo clarified Federal priorities in states liberalizing cannabis policies and tasked U.S. attorneys with preventing the following: cannabis sales to minors, illegal cartel activity, interstate trafficking of cannabis, drugged driving, any detriments to public health, and violence or accidents involved with the cannabis trade (Southall & Healy, 2013). The memo also contended that states with established and effective regulatory structures should manage growers, distributors, or sellers regardless of the size of operation and, therefore, do not warrant Federal intervention (Cole, 2013).[73]

Most recently, the 2018 Sessions Memo reversed the Ogden and Cole memos. The Sessions Memo reclaims the right of the Justice department to uphold the CSA irrespective of State laws. The language of the memo does not delineate between medical and recreational programs or players acting within, or outside, state programs.[74] [75]

Those in Congress that support the right of states to conduct medical cannabis programs have been able to offer some protection from the ebb and flow of the DEA's memos via the 2014 Rohrabacher–Farr Amendment (renamed Rohrabacher-Blumenauer when Farr retired). Attempts to pass such an amendment began in 2001, but did not succeed until 2014 as part of an omnibus spending bill. The Amendment does not change Federal cannabis legislation, rather denies funding to the Justice Department to interfere with state medical cannabis programs. The Amendment must be renewed annually, and (to date) Congress has been able to maintain a check in balance against the DEA via amendments to appropriations bills presently.

Industrial Hemp Cannabis

In 2004, the United States Court of Appeals, Ninth Circuit, decided in favor of Hemp Industries Association (HIA) vs. the DEA. This decision effectively legalized the import and distribution of products derived from non-psychoactive hemp plants (industrial hemp) because the court argued non-psychoactive hemp is not included in Schedule I.[76] Industrial hemp products could be imported and distributed, but industrial hemp was still illegal to grow in the United States without the authority of the DEA.

Under Section 7606 of the Agricultural Act of 2014 (2014 Farm Bill), the U.S. House of Representatives passed an amendment that defined *industrial hemp* as distinct from *marijuana* in that it is a cannabis plant that has less than 0.3 percent tetrahydrocannabinol, THC—a cannabinoid in cannabis associated with a more significant psychotropic, "high inducing" effect. The 2014 Farm Bill created a mechanism for states to pursue a pilot program to investigate the efficacy of hemp for industrial purposes.[77] This has allowed the production, research, and sale of industrial hemp products without the authority of the DEA (but under state-authorized mechanisms).

Similar to the debate over state medical and recreational cannabis programs, the DEA pushed back on industrial hemp programs, particularly as they pertain to the production and dispensing of cannabidiol (CBD). CBD is associated with a variety of health benefits (most notably its anti-inflammatory properties) and products. In 2016, the DEA published a final rule establishing a new drug code for cannabis extract which includes, but is not limited to, CBD oil.[78] The justification of the new code was to remain up to

45

date with international drug control treaties administered through the United Nations. The DEA argued they did not add CBD oil to the CSA; rather, they clarified existing definitions of marihuana and marihuana-derived products as it pertains to the Act. The crux of the DEA's argument was twofold. They deem any compounds derived from non-stem and non-stalk parts of the marihuana plant controlled substances. Since CBD is derived mainly from the flower and resinous leaves of the marihuana plant, they deem CBD a controlled substance. Hemp Industries Association argued the definition of marihuana under the CSA was different than that of cannabis, and that neither cannabis nor CBD were defined as controlled substances under the CSA. HIA argued that the 2014 Farm Bill's definition of industrial hemp as cannabis with .3 percent or less THC content was the rule of law.

The Hemp Industries Association filed suit against the DEA regarding the code creation, but the case was decided in favor of the DEA on procedural grounds, not the merits of the case. In their ruling; however, the judges made clear that CBD outside of the 2014 Farm Bill Industrial Hemp Pilot Research Programs was illegal.

The 2014 Farm Bill created a federally legal mechanism for CBD processing and dispensing. The 2014 Farm Bill defined industrial hemp cannabis away from cannabis as "marihuana" under the CSA and legalized cultivation, processing, and sale of any part of the industrial hemp plant, including CBD, as long as it is through state sanctioned pilot research programs. CBD products produced under a state sanctioned industrial hemp pilot research program with a regulatory framework that covers cultivation processing, sale, and import/export of industrial hemp are legal in the United States. Internal DEA memos support this. What the DEA maintains, and what is legally true, is that CBD production and sale outside of industrial hemp pilot research programs is not legal. The CSA's definition of "marihuana" cannabis includes any derivatives of the "marihuana" plant—including CBD. The 2014 Farm Bill trumps the CSA, but in order to garner the protections, operation within the framework of a state sanctioned pilot research program is required.

The pending 2018 Farm Bill includes an industrial hemp provision which would solidify that industrial hemp is separate from marijuana and thus the CSA. Where the legality of CBD will land with the passing of the 2018 Farm Bill is still a gray area.

* For the most recent discussions of the political landscapes of cannabis, please visit the blog section at www.phytopharmd.com

Section 2:
Cannabis Science

Chapter 7: Botany

Cannabis is a member of the Cannabaceae family. The Cannabaceae family is a diverse family made up of at least ten genera, as well as over 150 different species. These flowering plants are found throughout most of the world where tropical and temperate weather exists. Cannabaceae ranges from large trees and vines to herbaceous plants and can be annual or perennial. Celtis is the largest genus in the family with over 100 species. Cannabaceae plants tend to be dioecious, meaning they have a separate plant for male and female flowers. Their flowers are not usually showy (no corollas and only a small calyx), and the plants are frequently wind pollinated. The male flower is long while the female counterpart is compact.

Cannabis is an annually flowering dicot that can grow up to fifteen feet tall. Pairs of leaves grow from each node in early growth phases (opposite arrangement) and transition to a single leaf per node (alternate arrangement) as it matures. The leaves are palmately compound (shaped like the palm of a hand) with serrated leaflets. Plants typically have seven to nine leaflets, although some will have more depending on the species, growing inputs, and variety type. C. indica and C. sativa are short-day/long-night flowering plants. C. ruderalis appears to be autoflowering and is unaffected by photoperiod.

Typically, Cannabis is dioecious, meaning male and female reproductive organs are on separate plants, but it can produce monoecious plants, where the male and female flowers form on the same plant. Stressors, like the use of chemical treatments or a harsh environment, increase the likelihood of producing what is commonly referred to as a "hermaphrodite."

The male flowers form as panicles, loose branching clusters like oat, and produce five stamens that droop downward. Male plants flower one to two weeks earlier than female plants. Female cannabis produces a fruit called an achene, known to most as a cannabis seed. Female flowers form as racemes: separate flowers attached by short equal stalks at equal distances along a central stem.

51

Females have a prominent calyx—a green structure that protects its reproductive organs. Protruding out from the short calyx is a small hair called a pistil where the ovary, style, and stigma are contained. Female flowers on cannabis produce more trichomes than their male counterparts. Trichomes are responsible for deterring predators and protecting the plant from wind damage, potential fungal blooms, and damaging solar radiation. The stickiness of trichomes aid in pollen collection. From a medical and recreational consumption standpoint, the trichomes' most important attribute to cannabis is the production of phytochemicals such as cannabinoids and terpenes.

Cannabis species taxonomy is debated. The most prevalent method of delineating cannabis into sub-categories is based on a combination of plant structure, growing characteristics, and trends in consumption derived effects. Such categorization reduces the spectrum of strains to three categories: indica, sativa, or hybrid. In broad terms, indica plants are shorter, more dense, possess wider leaves, and have a denser flower structure. Indica plants are a heartier variety acclimated to cooler and higher altitude climates. They tend to elicit a more sedating effect often referred to as a "body high." Indica strains were primarily grown for their psychotropic effects. Indica-dominant plants are described to:

- Have maintained their origins closer to Central Asia
- Have shorter growth cycles
- Produce broader leaves
- Grow shorter and more robust
- Produce an intoxicating effect that is more sedative and full-body

Common Indica-dominant landrace strains are:

- Afghani
- Hindu Kush
- Ketama
- Lashkar Gah
- Pakistan Valley

Sativa plants tend to be taller and less dense, with longer/ skinnier leaves and flower structures. They are more prone to having difficulty with inclimate environments. Sativas tend to elicit a more cerebral high ("head-high") that is characterized as energizing rather than sedating. Historically, sativa plants were used for industrial use rather than as an intoxicant. Sativa-dominant plants are described to:

- Originate in Southeast Asia, Africa, and the Americas
- Have longer growth cycles
- Produce skinnier leaves
- Grow taller and thinner
- Produce an intoxicating effect that is more uplifting and heady

Common Sativa-dominant landrace strains are:

- Acapulco Gold
- Colombian Gold
- Durban Poison
- Kilimanjaro
- Malawi
- Panama Red
- South African Kwazulu
- Thai

Pure indica and sativa strains are no longer commonplace. Modern breeding has created myriad strains of cannabis combining indica and sativa characteristics. These strains are referred to as hybrids. They are bred for a variety of reasons including improved production outcome (increased yield, higher phytochemical content, and decreased propensity toward disease) and desired consumption effect.

Popular Indica-dominant hybrid strains are:

- Grandaddy Purple
- Bubba Kush
- Northern Lights
- White Rhino
- Super Skunk

Popular Sativa-dominant hybrid strains are:

- Jack Herer
- Super Lemon Haze
- Strawberry Cough
- Maui Wowie
- Candyland

Popular hybrid strains showing balanced sativa/indica attributes:

- Blue Dream
- Girl Scout Cookies
- OG Kush
- White Widow
- Gorilla Glue

Ruderalis is either another category of cannabis or a wild/ weeded offshoot of sativa. It historically grew wild in the Northern Himalayas, Northeastern Europe, and Midwestern United States. It is shorter, with a larger stem-than-leaf ratio. It is also more resistant to mold/mildew/pests and contains virtually no THC. When bred with sativas and indicas, it can produce autoflowering hybrids.

With few genetically pure strains today, and almost all medical and recreational cannabis strains being categorized as hybrids, there is a shifting focus in categorization of cannabis strains based on sativa/ indica delineations toward descriptions based on the phytochemical compositions of individual strains.

Chapter 8: Phytochemistry

Phytochemicals are biologically active chemical compounds produced through primary or secondary metabolism in plants in order to help the plant grow and/or protect itself from disease and pests.[79] [80] The term phytochemical includes both nutritional and non-nutritional compounds found in a plant; however, the term is generally used to refer to the non-essential nutrients and compounds in a plant.[81] Essential nutrients are compounds the human body can't make (or makes, but doesn't produce enough of) that are required for normal human body functioning. When considering the entirety of the plant (roots, stalk, leaves, seeds, and flowers), the phytochemical makeup of cannabis is quite profound.

Essential Nutrients

The known categories of essential nutrients for humans are:

- Water
- Calories (energy) from protein, carbohydrate, or fat
- 8-10 essential amino acids
- Essential fatty acids
- 13 vitamins
- 16-20 minerals[82]

A fresh cannabis plant is eighty percent water. Cannabis calories can be derived from protein, fats, and sugars. Cannabis seeds contain around 30% oil and about 25% protein. Thirty-three different fatty acids have been found in cannabis seed oil.[83] Polyunsaturated fatty acids account for 80% of cannabis seed oil. The proteins contained in cannabis seeds (mainly edestin and albumin) are highly nutritional in the form of easily digestible essential amino acids. [84] [85] The cannabis plant contains many sugars including thirteen monosaccharides, two disaccharides, five polysaccharides, and sugar alcohols. In addition, cannabis is a source for cyclitols. Fresh juice of the cannabis plant is a good source of vitamins, nutrients, protein, oil and insoluble fiber. Cannabis juice is rich in vitamin K, and eighteen elements have been found in cannabis including essential minerals sodium, potassium, calcium, magnesium, iron, copper, manganese, and zinc.[86]

Phytochemicals

All other biologically active chemical compounds produced by plants are considered non-essential nutrient, or non-nutrient phytochemicals. Despite their non-essential categorization, non-nutrient phytochemicals have been found to provide protection for human health.[87]

Cannabinoids

Phytochemical cannabinoids are chemical compounds found in cannabis that bind to receptors in the human body (See Chapter 10: Endocannabinoid System). There are currently over 100 known cannabinoids, though most of them have yet to be independently studied and fully characterized. Two of the better known cannabinoids are tetrahydrocannabinol (THC) and cannabidiol (CBD). THC is well known for the psychotropic/euphoric high it produces due to its activity as a partial agonist of CB1 receptors.[88] CBD is known for its anti-inflammatory,[89] anti-anxiety,[90] and seizure-reducing properties[91] with a reduced psychotropic effect. CBD is also a negative allosteric modulator on CB1 receptors[92] and a weak antagonist of CB2 receptors.[93] CBD is not as psychoactive as THC but does have a significant sedative effect at higher doses.

Other cannabinoids, while less studied, are also known to have therapeutic effects. Cannabigerol (CBG) is known for its antibacterial, anti-tumor, and sedative effects. Cannabinol (CBN) is the result of the oxidative process that occurs when THC is exposed to oxygen and heat; it can result from aging, exposure to sun, or overheating of THC products. While individual cannabinoids have different properties, their effect on the body is greater when different cannabinoids are combined than when they are used in isolation.[94] This synergistic interaction is commonly referred to as the "entourage effect" in the cannabis industry.

Some examples of cannabinoids found in cannabis and their associated benefits are:

- THC: generally the most abundant cannabinoid in cannabis, causing the most psychotropic effects
  - analgesic, appetite stimulant, antiemetic, antispasmodic
- THCa: main constituent in raw cannabis converting to Δ9-THC when heated (decarboxylated)
  - anti-inflammatory, anti epileptic, anti-proliferative
- THCv: minor cannabinoid found in only some strains of cannabis
  - anorectic, anti-epileptic, anti-diabetic, bone-stimulant
- CBN: mildly psychoactive cannabinoid that is produced from the degradation of THC
  - analgesic, antispasmodic, anti-somnia
- CBD: rather than an "on/off" or "lock and key" receptor mechanism, CBD modifies the receptiveness of endocannabinoid receptors and also appears to interact elsewhere in the body
  - analgesic, anti-inflammatory, appetite stimulant, antiemetic, intestinal anti-prokinetic, anxiolytic, antipsychotic, antiepileptic, antispasmodic, immunosuppressive, anti-diabetic, neuroprotective, antipsoriatic, anti-ischemic, antibacterial, anti-proliferative, bone-stimulant
- CBDa: CBD's form prior to decarboxylation
  - anti-inflammatory, anti-proliferative
- CBDv: non-psychoactive cannabinoid similar in structure to CBD
  - antiepileptic
- CBG: non-psychoactive cannabinoid
  - analgesic, anti-inflammatory, anti-bacterial, anti-fungal, anti-proliferative, bone-stimulant
- CBGa: CBG's form prior to decarboxylation
  - anti-inflammatory
- CBC: second most prevalent cannabinoid in cannabis produced through an enzymatic process converting CBGa to

CBCa, which then makes CBC when heated
- o analgesic, anti-inflammatory, anti-bacterial, anti-proliferative, bone-stimulant
- CBCa: CBC's form prior to decarboxylation
  - o anti-bacterial, anti-fungal

Terpenes

Terpenes are chemical compounds produced in plants that contribute to the plants' flavors and smells. Terpenes protect cannabis from environmental stressors such as excess moisture, mold, penetrating sun, and pests. Terpenes can also attract beneficials (helpful insects such as ladybugs). Like cannabinoids, terpenes interact with a multitude of receptors in the body.[95] Many of the benefits associated with essential oils are due to their high terpene contents. Two common terpenes in cannabis are alpha-pinene and D-linalool (also found in pine trees and lavender, respectively). Alpha-pinene has demonstrated anti-inflammatory,[96] bronchodilating,[97] and antibiotic[98] properties. Of special interest to cannabis researchers is alpha-pinene's ability to inhibit the breakdown of acetylcholine, which mitigates the short-term memory degradation associated with THC.[99] D-linalool has been shown to have anticonvulsant,[100] anxiety-reducing,[101] and sedative effects.[102] D-linalool also seems to have local anesthetic effects comparable to that of procaine and menthol,[103] which would be relevant in topical applications of cannabis.

Some terpenes found in cannabis, with their aroma/flavor, effect/medical value, and an example of each strain are:

- Myrcene: tropical and earthy; analgesic, anti-inflammatory, and antibiotic (Pure Kush)
- Limonene: citrus; antifungal, antibacterial properties, and anticarcinogenic (Super Lemon Haze)
- Pinene: pine; expectorant, bronchodilator, anti-inflammatory, and local antiseptic (Jack Herer)
- Eucalyptol: mint; pain relief and improved concentration (ChemDawg)
- Terpineol: floral; sedative (White Rhino)

- Borneol: mint; combat fatigue, stress, and illness (Diamond Girl)
- Caryophyllene: pepper; anti-inflammatory and analgesic (Super Silver Haze)
- Linalool: lavender; anti-anxiety and sedative (Grape Ape)

Flavonoids

Flavonoids play a role in the color and aroma of flowers to assist in attracting pollinators and are involved in seed and spore germination.[104] During growth, they help the plant filter light[105] and protect them from mold, mildew, and pests.[106] Flavonoids are suspected to play an influential role in the effect that cannabis produces but are currently the least studied of the compounds in cannabis. They are a key area of investigation for scientists studying the health effects of plant consumption and have been studied for their antiviral,[107] antibacterial,[108] anti-inflammatory,[109] neuroprotective and regenerative,[110] anti-oxidative,[111] and anti-cancer effects.[112] There is significant need for additional studies on how flavonoids interact with cannabinoids and terpenes.

Others

Very little is known about the beneficial potential of other lesser known cannabis phytochemicals such as alkanes, amines, phenols, alcohols, aldehydes, ketones, acids, esters, and lactones. These additional constituents further enhance and differentiate flavors and aromas, and fruit and vegetable research is showing their contribution to various health benefits.

Influencing Phytochemical Composition

Factors that affect the essential nutrients and phytochemical composition of plants include genetic makeup, degree of maturity, environmental conditions, postharvest handling, and storage.[113] In addition:

> Although volatile compounds are synthesized via a few major biochemical pathways, various forms of enzymatic

modifications such as hydroxylations, acetylations, and methylations, add to the diversity of emitted volatiles by increasing their volatility at the final step of their formation [124,125]. An important step in the biosynthetic pathway of aroma compounds is the availability of primary recursor substrates, including fatty acids and amino acids...[114]

Variations in type and amount of base building blocks and catalysts influence the trajectory of plant composition. Furthermore, accessibility to various compounds in plants occur at different stages of plant development and harvest. This array of factors influencing cannabis production is an emerging area of increased attention and research.

Chapter 9: Production

Cultivation

Before a person starts to cultivate cannabis, whether for their own use or for commercial production, there are many factors to be considered. Cannabis can be grown outdoors, in a greenhouse, or indoors. Each environment presents its own benefits and obstacles. If grown indoors, there are multiple lighting options to choose from that will vary in cost, yield, and quality. These options, among others, should be reviewed for cost-effectiveness before beginning the process.

Outdoor Cultivation

Factors affecting outdoor cannabis cultivation include: climate, soil quality, water availability, light cycles, and security. While cannabis is adaptive, and certain strains are able to withstand a greater degree of severity in temperature and moisture, cannabis thrives in climates that have sustained temperate environments. Considering the location of feral cannabis historically and the locations in which it thrives today offers insight into the ideal outdoor setting for cannabis cultivation:

> Feral *Cannabis* populations are found growing in temperate climates at northern latitudes. These are usually characterized as warm continental regions with spring and early summer rains, followed by a dry cool autumn and accompanied by the widely fluctuating day length (photoperiod) afforded by more northern (and more southern) latitudes; indeed feral *Cannabis* only flourishes in this narrow climate niche. The vegetation cover most favourable for *Cannabis* is temperate-climate upland open woodland growing in valleys with alluvial soil deposits and slopes for drainage with sufficient sunlight and summer rainfall. Suitable regions would have had moist temperate conditions during glaciations without being so near the equator as to lose short-day flowering response and cold hardiness.[115]

Typically, cannabis grown outdoors is planted in soil. Depending on the ground soil quality, some outdoor cannabis cultivators import supplemented soil (and/or provide added nutrients to ground soil) to improve cultivation outcomes. Sustainable farming practices are also being applied to cannabis cultivation. Some growers, such as Green Source Gardens in Oregon, achieve a healthy biological soil ecosystem through poly-culture gardens where diverse plant species include dynamic accumulators that increase aroma, vigor, potency, and overall plant health. Their methods are rooted in bio-dynamics, permaculture, and indigenous agriculture.[116]

Like any other plant, if cannabis is watered too little or too much it will not grow to healthy yields. Each cannabis plant needs between twenty to forty gallons of water during the growing season. This number will depend on the soil type, amount of sun, and strain being grown. Impurities in the water supply (heavy metals or pesticides) can be absorbed by the plant and find their way into the final product.

The amount of sunlight cannabis needs is growth-stage dependant. Generally, cannabis plants grow during the long days of summer and then begin to flower as days begin to shorten. Certain strains have adapted, or been bred, to withstand extended or shortened light periods. Cultivators able to grow multiple harvests, in a year are tuned in to how seasonal light availability influences cultivation.

Even with the correct climate, soil, water, and sunlight, pests and wildlife can disrupt successful cultivation. Netting, root and canopy fencing, beneficial and/or predatory insects, poli-cropping, and herbal repellents are natural approaches to protecting a garden. Chemical herbicides, fungicides, insecticides, miticides, and rodenticides are sometimes used in cultivation techniques. The use of these chemicals are potentially harmful to the farmer, surrounding ecosystem, and consumer. Many states regulate the chemicals that can be used.

Greenhouse Cultivation

Growing cannabis in a greenhouse environment offers many of the benefits of both indoor and outdoor cultivation. The structure itself mitigates some propensity for disease and pests. Greenhouse growers commonly use soil as the growing medium and the power of the natural sun, but in a more climate controllable setting. Low velocity intake, exhaust fans, and insulation can help maintain the temperature, humidity, and air quality of the growing environment. Light can be altered in a greenhouse; supplemental lighting can be used in winter months to provide longer light cycles and light deprivation techniques can be used to keep plants in a flowering state.

Indoor Cultivation

Growing cannabis indoors under the right conditions can increase crop quality and yield. Indoor cannabis cultivation allows for a controlled environment, which eliminates or reduces some of the variables associated with outdoor or greenhouse growing. Indoor cultivation, whether in-home or commercial, must be vented to ensure proper humidity and temperature controls. Indoor growing avoids the array of outdoor pests and wildlife that can harm plants and relies on the use of powerful artificial lights to replicate the effects of the sun, allowing for complete control over light cycles and flowering phases. There are a variety of indoor growing methods: soil, drip irrigation, coco coir or rockwool, hydroponics, and mediumless aeroponics. One of the biggest negative consequences of indoor growing is the increased consumption of energy due to artificial lighting and HVAC demands. Some indoor growers are working to reduce energy consumption by equipping facilities with renewable energy sources such as solar or wind power, choosing lights that require less energy, and installing environmental control systems with more sustainable designs in growing facilities.

Plant Selection

Choosing appropriate strains based on the cultivation environment can help maximize yield.

Outdoor Cultivation

As described previously, cannabis grows with more success in specific climates. However, cannabis is a hearty plant and has spread with a great deal of success all over the world from its origins in Central Asia. Hardiness zones—as they relate to length of grow season, average precipitation, day length, average temperature, altitude, and soil quality—will influence which strains have propensity for increased success.

The hardiness zone will also define the number of outdoor harvests and yield potential to be expected per year. It is possible to manipulate an outdoor environment to increase potential harvests and yields. This can be done through additional watering or soil drainage, adding lighting or creating light deprivation, choosing shaded or full-sun locations, and adding nutrients to the soil.

Specific strains tend to do better in various outdoor climates, so choosing zone-specific strains will also help your success. Here are some suggested strains for specific climates:

- Tropical – Super Silver Haze or Bob Marley Sativa
- Mediterranean – Jack Herer or Blueberry
- Subtropical – Candy Kush or White Widow
- Arid – Durban Poison or Yoruba Nigeria
- Temperate – Holland's Hope or Light of Jah
- Continental – Northern Lights or Amnesia Haze
- Subarctic – Lemon Haze Auto or Purple Power

Greenhouse and Commercial Cultivation

When choosing strains for greenhouse and indoor cultivation, the biggest issues to account for are the height and girth of each plant. The space available in a greenhouse or facility can influence strain choice, as various plants grow to different sizes. Growing techniques, such as super cropping and no-veg aeroponic growing, can open the possibilities of growing notoriously tall plants more easily indoors.

New greenhouse and indoor technologies can easily maintain room-specific climate controlled settings. The degree to which a greenhouse or indoor facility is controlled will also influence the strains success. For example, if it is not possible to keep the environment cool enough, strains notoriously more successful in warmer climates are better choices.

If grow techniques are being deployed in facilities that afford more range of strains, the last set of attributes to consider is each strain's resistance to disease and pests, yield potential, and potency test results. As the commercial sale of seeds and plants increases and genetics stabilize, informative label information is more readily available to help with such choices.

Breeding

Cannabis has gradually co-evolved with humans for thousands of years as food, fiber, and medicine, but it is within the last fifty years that humans have played a more active role in selective breeding and created the variety of cultivars present today. In cannabis breeding, genetic information is transferred from the pollen of the male plant to the pistil of the female plant. Growers will attempt to combine the best traits of their best strains to maximize yield, alter the phytochemical composition, or simply to better mold a strain to its environment.

Genotypes are the encoded genetic material of a strain, while the phenotype is the physical manifestation of these genetics as the plant responds to its environment (grows). As with all breeding, dominant and recessive genes play a role. Dominant genes will be more pronounced, whereas the recessive genes will only be displayed when matched up with another recessive gene.

The first step in breeding is choosing the right parents to achieve the desired results. Two common methodologies of cannabis breeding are "backcrossing" and "F1 hybrids". Backcrossing is a technique that consists of a strain being crossed back into one of its own parents. This type of breeding creates strains with more stability in the desired characteristics from the parents that will pass to future generations. When using this technique, the recessive traits will get passed down at a higher rate. To avoid this, backcrossing should not be executed multiple times.

F1 hybrids are first generation crosses of two unique strains. These hybrids are where genetic diversity is created in cannabis and predictability is traded for an increased potential of finding the next great strain. Once a great F1 has been found, the two parent plants can continue to be crossed to produce more of that type; although, to reliably recreate the same combination of genetics you will have to resort to the aforementioned backcrossing technique.

After choosing the plants for hybridizing, males and females are isolated. This reduces the chance of early pollination. Once they have been separated and flowering has occurred, the male pollen sacs will open, and pollen will be released. Collecting pollen from the males can be done by harvesting the entirety of the pollen sacs or shaking pollen on a plate every day for a couple of weeks. If pollen is being stored long term, it can be placed in the freezer for an extended period of time. Saving the prized males in vegetative growth and taking cuttings to flower when pollen is needed is another way to keep desired male genetics consistent. Female flowers are usually ready to be pollinated 2-4 weeks after the pistils have started to grow. If pollinated too early, seeds will not develop. If done too late, the seeds will not get time to mature and will not be viable. Closing of all ventilation and sterilizing of clothing are crucial to stop cross contamination of different pollens. Cannabis pollen is very small and can travel great distances before finding a female flower. There are several ways in which growers pollinate their plants when they want to create seeds. Hand pollination uses tools like paint brushes, matches, or cotton swabs to dab the female pistils with the pollen.

Another method is to close off an entire room of females and pollinate the entire room. Some breeders will leave fans and ventilation active and place male flowering plants in the rooms with the females that they want to be pollinated so that natural wind pollination takes place. Alternatively, some growers prefer to selectively pollinate just a few plants, branches, or individual flowers instead of all the plants in their grow. In order to do this, they place a paper bag over the flowers that have been hand pollinated for about 5 days to ensure that they do not spread pollen to other flowers. Once a plant has been fertilized, some may prefer a boost in fertilizers for maximum production. Seeds are ready to collect when they start pushing out of their calyx; this happens several weeks after pollination. Ideal storage for seeds is a cool, dry place, but seeds should not be placed in the freezer.

The most important part of a breeding program is labeling and taking excellent data in order to properly track desired outcomes. Through this practice, breeders are able to learn from the crosses that have been made and may apply their gathered data accordingly to future breeding methods. Breeding for optimal traits can be accomplished by incorporating this structured practice into any breeding technique. It is very important to continue evaluating throughout the entire growing cycle, curing process, and final product stage. Serious breeders even have new plants sent to multiple labs for testing. The more that is recorded and observed, the easier it is to determine nuanced attributes like which traits are dominant and recessive.

Propagation

Cannabis can be propagated either sexually or asexually, and different situations and goals will determine which is preferential to any given grower. Sexual propagation is achieved by taking pollen from a male and having it come into contact with a pistil on a female plant; and ultimately, this process forms seeds. Asexual propagation can be done by taking vegetative parts from either male or female plants and grafting, cutting (cloning), or tissue culturing. Asexual propagation is a more recent phenomenon in cannabis, cultivation predominantly done with cuttings or "clones" from a mother plant during its vegetative phase. Both sexual and asexual propagation have their place in modern day cannabis growing.

"Cracking" Seeds

Sexual (seed) propagation is still the most commonly used method of producing cannabis. A cannabis seed can be kept viable for years if stored properly; this has historically allowed for widespread distribution among trade routes. Not only is sexual propagation advantageous because of its storage and trade benefits, but this type of breeding allows for the genes of both parents to combine to express a unique combination of this shared genetic code. Every seed is essentially a new plant with an entirely new set of characteristics. This high variance has opened up and expanded the complex cannabinoid, terpenoid, and flavonoid possibilities. Sexual propagation gives cannabis plants a more robust growth form and more vigorous root system. Plants grown from seed will develop taproots, which aid in stability and are especially desirable in soil, as they travel further down in search of water and nutrients.

Feminized seeds are a result of modifications to the normal seed process which genetically modify the seeds to contain no male chromosomes. This ensures that the plant grown will only have the female flowering organs ensuring that pollination does not occur. These seeds are created by inducing male flowers to grow on a female plant by treating the plant with specific chemicals. Once the female plant produces pollen sacs, the pollen from these sacs is used to pollinate itself and other females of other cultivars. This results in a seed that only has the female chromosomes; no male organs are produced. In some instances, feminized seeds can produce hermaphrodite plants, which will (unexpectedly) produce pollen. This can potentially pollinate an entire harvest. Sexual propagation does require more energy, nutrients, labor, and cost because of the added time it takes to reach harvest.

Cloning

Vegetative propagation, done by taking cuttings from the plant prior to it entering the flowering state, has been used with success throughout the modern cannabis industry. By taking cuttings of cannabis, one can replicate a genotype into numerous genetically identical plants, typically referred to as "clones." Although different phenotypes can be expressed in the clones depending on the environmental stressors they respond to, they still share an identical genotype. Cloning is the quickest path to harvest, as it cuts down on the grow time significantly and removes the need for sexing. Healthy, robust mother plants yield about 70-100 cuttings each; working with 24 mother plants would produce about eight plants in a three week rotation to take cuttings from. A master propagator can produce 600 cuttings in one day, and large scale commercial producers use this method frequently. It is consistent, time-effective, and assists in giving the growers a regular schedule for lighting, nutrients, harvesting, drying and curing. Market requirements for specific strains can be more easily met by cloning plants that are in high need, thus supplying the demand in a shorter feedback loop.

Cloners of cannabis need to be vigilant about viruses, diseases, and long-term degradation of the strain. Viruses and diseases can be transferred from the parent plant to the cuttings. The cuttings need to be kept clean, and it is important to sterilize cutting tools between plants to avoid spreading diseases. The cuttings are susceptible to fungal infections and need to be treated with care. The debate is still out, but it is thought that taking clones long-term can lead to degradation of that strain, gradually producing less vigorous and potent plants. However, some growers will keep parent plants around for years, claiming little to no degradation of the strain.

Tissue Culture

The development of tissue culturing is giving growers a more sterile, consistent option when it comes to asexual propagation. Plant parts (seeds, leaves, stems, or roots) are placed in a sterile gel medium (derived from algae) that contains different combinations of sugars, plant growth hormones, and agar. This nutrient solution is what the new plants will grow out of and must be in a sterile environment. It is typically done in a lab under a HEPA hood vent to clear the air of outside influences like mold and fungi spores. Plants are often kept sealed in vitro (in glass) inside a large growing chamber that has optimal light, air, and temperature settings until they are large enough to be planted into the medium of choice. Propagating this way gives the growers exact replicas of the plant for high-efficiency production like cloning, but it also eliminates unwanted infections spreading. Tissue culturing allows for the replication of many plants from a single piece of a plant, as long as all genetic information needed is stored within. All of the plants started this way are free from disease and virus, making them risk-free for the grower. Proper setup can be expensive and techniques for tissue culturing cannabis are limited at this point. Experts in this field are hesitant to bring their skill sets into the cannabis industry because of current Federal illegality.

Grafting

Grafting is yet another method to asexually propagate cannabis. This is typically done on a small scale but could prove to be interesting for larger growers. Grafting gives the grower with limited space the ability to have multiple varieties on one parent plant. That way, the grower has access to different strains without taking up space. It could also prove beneficial for strains that will not root well in the cutting stage but may thrive if grafted onto a vigorous rootstock. As of now, grafting seems limited to only a handful of growers.

Harvest

Each cannabis producer has a unique approach to determining when a crop is ready to be harvested and move to the drying, trimming, and curing process. This section speaks to general practices rather than a set of specific techniques.

There are several visual indications that cannabis is ready to harvest. As the length of light exposure is reduced (the days become shorter), a transition will occur. This is true for both outdoor and indoor growing, with the notable exception of "auto-flowering" plants which have cannabis ruderalis genetics. Regardless of specifics, the buds should display more trichome coverage and become more voluminous as they mature. When the pistils start to turn color, the plant is getting close, but the truest indication of harvest time are the trichome heads themselves. Trichomes are resin glands that look like mushrooms up close.

Most growers use a jeweler's loupe or similar device that can magnify at least 60x, ideally with backlighting. The trichome heads will start translucent, then turn cloudy, and finally start to turn amber. There will be grower preference and strain specific preferences, but it is typically thought that cloudy heads will yield a more cerebral or invigorating effect while the amber heads indicate degradation into CBN and provide the classic body high "couchlock" effect. The trichomes will progress at different rates, so some ratio of cloud to amber heads will occur.

Harvesting begins with the removal of all the large fan leaves, which expedites the drying and trimming processes. One exception is in the case of an exceptionally dry environment. A very dry environment may dry the flower too quickly, and leaving some leaf material may help retain moisture. Limbs are cut into roughly two foot lengths and are often hung to dry.

Dry

Dry rooms maintain clean and sterile conditions, with minimal light, around 60 degrees and 50-60% humidity. Plants are hung upside down, often as single branches, to ensure that there is good airflow to prevent mold or mildew issues. The first half of plant water weight is removed within 48 hours to lower the chance of mold growth, and the drying phase is typically three to seven days in total. The pliability of the stem (bend vs. snap), sponginess of the bud, and aroma will all provide clues as to how dry the bud is. Over-drying cannabis impedes the ability to cure it properly.

Trim

Trimming can be done at any stage of drying, although it is typically done after the initial dry and before the cure. Trimming while cannabis is still moist will make the buds less brittle, but it will be harder to get out leaf material as it is still very resinous and sticks to the underlying bud. Trimming is traditionally done with trimming scissors, although there are increasing efforts being made to automate the process. The goal is to remove as much of the lower potency leaf material as possible, while minimizing the handling of the bud so as to not knock off valuable trichomes. Often there is a sorting of bud qualities and a collection of trim to be processed into myriad cannabis by-products.

Cure

Curing usually occurs after the initial drying phase and typically after the flower has been trimmed. It is ideal to leave cannabis in airtight containers (like glass jars) for one to six months, maintaining 60-65% humidity, minimal light, and a temperature of 60 degrees. The containers are "burped" daily initially, until the moisture has dropped off. Odor, sponginess, and stem pliability are indicators of continued drying and curing.

Packaging

Cannabis flower is stored like wine in a cool, dark place. Hermetically sealed containers that have been vacuum sealed and flushed with an inert gas like nitrogen to prevent oxidation are a common way to store cannabis. Glass is the best material to store cannabis in, but the general trend is food grade mylar bags.

Processing

Once cannabis has been cultivated, it is common practice to further process the cannabis flower into a concentrated extraction or infuse it into a food-grade substance (such as coconut oil). This has the benefit of increasing the relative levels of therapeutic compounds compared to inert compounds. There are numerous processes that can be used to do this, and the end result can be vaporized, smoked, eaten, or turned into many different products like topicals and transdermal patches.

Solventless - Mechanical Extraction

Many traditional methods of making hashish (or hash) use relatively simple mechanical processes to separate trichomes from the rest of the plant material. The kief collected in the bottom of a grinder could be considered the most basic form of concentrated cannabis as the trichomes have separated from the relatively less potent buds. Dry sift hash uses specific screen sizes to formalize this process and select different compounds. Ice water hash utilizes the mild solvent properties of water to assist in separating trichomes from the plant before running the solution through similar screens. Rosin is produced by applying heat and pressure to cured cannabis and squeezing out the desired compounds.

Food-grade Oil Infusion

To create the base material for edibles and other orally administered medications, a food grade oil and cannabis are heated over low heat (~200°F) to infuse the liquid with the desired compounds. The plant material is then filtered out. The infused oil can be placed into edible food products, capsules, or consumed directly. Infused food grade oils are used in topical applications as well.

Passive Alcohol Extraction

The "Rick Simpson Method" produces what has been widely considered the most medically efficacious product. This process produces a thick sap that is highly concentrated cannabis oil. The process involves soaking cannabis in alcohol, straining out the plant material, and then evaporating ALL of the alcohol over low heat.

Another passive alcohol extraction method is an alcohol tincture. Cannabis can be soaked in alcohol for an extended period of time. The resulting tincture can be consumed either directly or after diluting with water. The ratio of cannabis to alcohol is high enough that the alcohol presence is insufficient to contraindicate.

High-pressure-closed Loop Hydrocarbon Extraction

The most common way to produce vaporizable (dabable) extracts is with a high pressure "closed loop" process involving a solvent, such as butane or carbon dioxide (CO_2). The pressurized solvent is allowed to pass through the cannabis and pull compounds out of the plant material, and the compounds are later pulled back out of that solvent. The end consistency can be anywhere from a solid "shatter" to a gooey sap, depending on the ratio of crystalline cannabinoids to more viscous terpenes (among many other pertinent compounds). The equipment for this process tends to be more expensive, and the THC content (among other cannabinoids) of the resulting product is of particular emphasis.

Short-path Distillation

Once the initial extraction from cannabis is obtained, it can be put through further purification processes to isolate the constituent compounds. This process is often referred to as short path distillation and can result in isolated cannabinoids, terpenes, or a "High Terpene/ Cannabinoid Full Spectrum Extract" which denotes an extremely high level of purity while maintaining a more complete spectrum of compounds. Using the appropriate techniques, any desired molecule should be able to be isolated or recombined as necessary.

* For the most recent discussions on cannabis production, please visit the blog section at www.WholePlantTechnologies.com

Section 3:
Cannabis as Medicine

Chapter 10: Endocannabinoid System

The endocannabinoid system (ECS) is named for the plant that led to its discovery, but evolutionary evidence shows us that it had been a central component of human physiology for hundreds of millions of years before cannabis existed.[117,118] The ECS began to evolve in complex lifeforms 600 million years ago:

> …[it]plays a master-regulatory role in many physiological functions that humans may naturally wish to self-adjust, such as mood, appetite, memory, inflammation, muscle tone, pain perception, and stress management, in addition to other more subtle but equally validated functions such as neuroprotection, bone growth, immunity, tumor regulation, seizure threshold, gastrointestinal motility, and intraocular pressure, to name a few.[119]

Despite early evolution of the ECS and its central role in body function, the ECS was not discovered until 1992. Initially, cannabis derived cannabinoids were discovered in 1964 via the isolation of THC.[120] CBD was soon after isolated as well. Investigating THC's effect on the body led to the discovery of the ECS.

The ECS is made up of three main components: cannabinoid receptors, endogenous cannabinoids, and enzymes. The first cannabinoid receptor was found in 1988 and coined the CB1 receptor. A second receptor, the CB2, was found soon after.[121] Cannabinoid receptors are found on the cell surface and influence how messages are sent, received, and processed by cells in order to maintain a homeostatic (healthy/balanced) state.[122] CB1 receptors are most densely concentrated in the central nervous system (CNS), especially in areas of nociception (pain perception), short-term memory, and basal ganglia, but they are also found in the peripheral nerves, uterus, testes, bones, and most other body tissues. Due to their location in the CNS, CB1 receptors are responsible for the psychoactive effects of THC. CB2 receptors, in contrast, are mostly found in the periphery, often in conjunction with immune cells. They may also appear in the CNS, particularly under conditions of inflammation in association with microcytes.[123] CB1 and CB2 are the most common ECS receptors, although cannabinoids can bind to at least another eight receptors that are not part of the mainstream conception of the ECS.[124,125]

When cannabinoid receptors were discovered, scientists still did not know why they existed in the body. It was not until 1992 with the discovery of the first, and soon after second, endogenous cannabinoid discovery that scientists realized there was a complete endocannabinoid system in the body. Endogenous cannabinoids (endocannabinoids) are natural chemicals produced by the body to activate cannabinoid receptors. The first two endocannabinoids discovered were N-arachidonoyl-ethanolamine (AEA; anandamide) and 2-arachidonoylglycerol (2-AG). Anandamide and 2-AG are lipid-derived agonists that are made on demand from the lipid bilayer and degraded by membrane-associated enzymes, negating the need for vesicle storage.[126] To simplify this concept, imagine the endocannabinoids as water from the tap in your home. When you are thirsty or need water for another purpose, you turn the tap on and get the amount of water needed. When you are finished with the intended use of the water, if any is left, you pour it down the drain. Because of the ability to instantly obtain and discard water, you do not need to store it in containers in your home. This same concept applies to the endocannabinoids in our body.

Ananda is the Sanskrit word for "joy, bliss, or happiness."[127] Anandamide is often associated with the cannabis plant derived cannabinoid THC. While endocannabinoids and plant derived cannabinoids share commonalities, there is not a 1:1 replacement between endocannabinoids and plant derived cannabinoids. They all interact with cannabinoid receptors differently. Anandamide has a greater affinity to bind to the CB1 receptor compared to the CB2 receptor, but THC has a very low affinity to the CB2. 2-AG has a greater affinity to the CB2 receptor, but also engages with the CB1 receptor. Plant derived CBD has little affinity to bind to either the CB1 or CB2 receptor, but it does influence endocannabinoid receptor affinity and modulates several non-cannabinoid receptors.

Enzymes synthesize and degrade endocannabinoids. This is to say, enzymes jump-start (catalyze) the creation of endocannabinoids and conversely work to metabolize, or modify, endocannabinoids to negate their signaling effect. Anandamide and 2-AG are degraded by the enzymes fatty acid amide hydrolase (FAAH)[128] and monoacylglycerol lipase (MAGL),[129] respectively. Without these enzymes, endocannabinoid levels would not dissipate, and homeostasis would not be maintained. While the effects of cannabis plant derived cannabinoids on the ECS garners most of the attention, one of the most exciting areas of ECS research is the potential to improve the body's own synthesis of endocannabinoids and also potential to slow degradation for prolonged beneficial effect via a better understanding of enzyme synthesis and degradation.[130]

The ECS is tasked with regulating multiple functions of the brain and body.

> ...[it] is one of the most important physiologic systems involved in establishing and maintaining human health. Endocannabinoids and their receptors are found throughout the body: in the brain, organs, connective tissues, glands, and immune cells. With its complex actions in our immune system, nervous system, and virtually all of the body's organs, the endocannabinoids are literally a bridge between body and mind. By understanding this system, we begin to see a mechanism that could connect brain activity and states of physical health and disease.[131]

The discovery of cannabis plant derived cannabinoids lead to the discovery of the ECS. Continued research on the interplay of cannabis plant derived cannabinoids and the ECS informs much of our understanding of cannabis-as-medicine. Cannabis interacts with the ECS, which is responsible for the promotion of homeostasis (balance) within various functions in the body. Cells require specific environments in order to function properly. An example of this is blood sugar. If a person's blood sugar is too high or too low, their cells can not properly perform the necessary functions. Through evolution, the human body has developed ways to ensure its various

79

processes remain in homeostasis. Through research, it has been discovered that cannabis derived cannabinoids can augment the ECS to relieve symptoms caused by a suppressed ECS and/or due to a disease state which shares symptoms in body functions the ECS can help to regulate.

Chapter 11: Research and Findings

As was described in earlier sections, the DEA's schedule I delineation of cannabis as a drug "with no currently accepted medical use and a high potential for abuse"[132] impedes the accessibility to research cannabis. Even in states where medical or recreational cannabis is allowed, research barriers exist. Despite these hurdles, there is clinical evidence that cannabis works as medicine.

The National Academies of Science, Engineering, and Medicine (NASEM) published a comprehensive cannabis review in 2017 that included 10,000 articles published since 1999. No case studies or conference reports were included in the articles reviewed. The study found substantial evidence of cannabis efficacy in treating chronic pain, chemotherapy-induced nausea and vomiting, and patient-reported multiple-sclerosis spasticity. The study also found some level of efficacy for increased appetite and decreased weight loss in HIV/AIDS, improved clinician-measured multiple sclerosis spasticity, improved symptoms of Tourette syndrome, decreased anxiety from generalized anxiety disorder, and decreased symptoms of PTSD.[133] The academy filtered out all case studies and conference reports for this review; however, there is value in examining case studies in aggregate for extrapolating beneficial effects and potential drug and condition interactions.

Below is a review of findings for various disease states patients tend to consider cannabis medicine for as a therapeutic option. This is not a comprehensive list of disease states that cannabis can treat as this primer is intended to be an introduction to medical cannabis, and subsequent editions of this primer will work to cover more.

Pain

The NASEM review found pain relief to be the most common reason patients sought treatment with medical cannabis. The National Institute on Drug Addiction reports more than 90 people die from opioid overdoses in the United States every day. When factoring in the cost of hospitalization, treatment, and criminal proceedings, the United States has an economic burden of over $78 billion per year on prescription opioids alone, according to CDC estimates.[134] States that have legalized medical cannabis have seen an almost 25% reduction in opioid overdose deaths.[135] These states have also seen a 23% reduction in hospitalizations due to opioid dependence or abuse and a 13% decrease in opioid overdose.[136] These results show the need for further investigation into the use of cannabis as a pain relief medication.[137]

The pathway used by medical cannabis to treat pain is a similar, but different, pathway than that which is used by opioid medications. Animal data shows the potential for medical application of cannabis to treat pain ranging from as effective as morphine to up to ten times as effective as other opioid medications. However, so far, studies in human population have not reproduced the same results as of yet. The major limitation to these studies tends to be psychoactive side effects in the medical cannabis patients.[138,139] Taking cannabis with opioids gives a heightened response to both medications, meaning a lower dose of each can be taken, leading to fewer side effects experienced by the patient.[140] Lowering the dose of opioids the patient is taking can decrease the chance of hospitalization due to accidental overdose and the chance of overdose related death

It has been shown that after exposure to pain, endocannabinoid levels are increased. This indicates that the endocannabinoid system plays a role in the modulation and perception of pain signaling. These increased endocannabinoid levels lead to the release of gamma-aminobutyric acid (GABA—an inhibitory neurotransmitter) in the periaqueductal gray matter, the rostral ventromedial medulla, and the superficial dorsal horn. These are the areas of the brain known for modulating pain stimuli.[141]

THC is the most known cannabinoid for having the ability to attenuate pain. This is due to the effect THC has on the CB1 receptors located in the brain. With these receptors being primarily located in the brain, this also causes THC to have more psychoactive side effects associated with its use. CBD interacts with CB2 receptors located in the periphery. CBD works as an analgesic and an anti-inflammatory by blocking the release of inflammatory mediators. By activating receptors peripherally, and not in the brain, CBD is able to provide pain relief without the risk of psychoactive adverse effects.[142] There is limited evidence that long term activation of CB1 receptors can lead to anti-inflammatory response.[143]

Chemotherapy Induced N/V

A common side effect of cancer treating medication regimens is nausea and vomiting. More than half the patients receiving this form of treatment will experience the side effect. This is due to the chemotherapeutic agents interacting with receptors in the gastrointestinal tract (GI) and the brain. Typically, nausea (the feeling of needing to vomit) is harder to treat than vomiting. Often, medical therapy will succeed in eliminating or reducing the amount of vomiting, but the nausea will be unaffected. Nausea is often reported as more bothersome because the feeling is constant whereas vomiting tends to occur at discrete times or patterns.[144]

Nausea/vomiting can start to occur within hours to days of receiving treatment, depending on which chemotherapeutic agent was received.[145] This can lead to declining quality of life in cancer patients, with patients often reporting the nausea and vomiting to be the most difficult side effect to deal with.[146] Patients that experience prolonged nausea and vomiting are more prone to electrolyte imbalances, weakness, and pneumonia. These concomitant conditions could prohibit the patient from staying on schedule with the chemotherapy regimens, further complicating their cancer treatment.[147]

In traditional pharmacy, there are three main treatments for chemotherapy induced nausea and vomiting. The first is 5-HT3 (serotonin) receptor antagonists. This category includes medications such as Zofran (ondansetron) and Kytril (granisetron). These drugs work on serotonin receptors located in the brain that cause nausea and vomiting.[148] By blocking this interaction, nausea and vomiting can be prevented. The second treatment option is dexamethasone, a corticosteroid. The mechanism for how dexamethasone helps to prevent acute and delayed nausea and vomiting is unknown; however, it has been shown to be an effective treatment.[149] The third treatment option is Emend (aprepitant). Aprepitant works by inhibiting the NK-1 neuroreceptor which affects the binding of Substance P. Substance P is a modulator that can induce nausea and vomiting when it interacts with NK-1 receptors in the gastrointestinal tract and the brain.[150]

Chemotherapeutic agents are separated into four categories based on their potential to cause nausea and vomiting. For patients with a chemotherapeutic drug that falls into the high category, the recommended prevention regimen consists of a serotonin receptor antagonist, dexamethasone, and Emend (aprepitant). Patients on a chemotherapeutic drug in the moderate category are treated with a serotonin receptor agonist and dexamethasone. Patients that fall into the low or minimal categories are treated with dexamethasone alone. Those in this category are unlikely to experience the nausea and vomiting side effects, but it is still encouraged to treat with dexamethasone to minimize the risk.[151]

The majority of studies available that detail the efficacy of cannabis for the treatment of nausea and vomiting have been performed in animal studies. What human data is available comes from small studies that are difficult to draw steadfast conclusions from. Despite the lack of human data, the FDA has approved Marinol (dronabinol), a synthetic version of THC, and Cesamet (nabilone), a synthetic medication similar to THC that activates CB1 receptors, for the treatment of chemotherapy induced nausea and vomiting.[152,153] With the approval of these medications, and the promising animal data, more human studies can be expected to show what effects cannabis will have on nausea and vomiting in the human population.

In animals, cannabis has been shown to be more effective than placebo and as, or more, effective than traditional medicine.[154,155] These studies have shown that CB1 receptors are located in the areas of the brain associated with nausea and vomiting and thus are viable targets for treatment.[156] The dorsal vagal complex contains both CB1 receptors and serotonin receptors (a common target for new anti-nausea medications). Cannabis is thought to reduce nausea and

84

vomiting by activating CB1 receptors and antagonizing serotonin receptors in this area via reduction of the release of serotonin. Interestingly, low doses of cannabis and ondansetron (a popular serotonin receptor antagonist antiemetic) that were ineffective when given separately were able to provide relief if given in conjunction.[157] Another cannabinoid found in cannabis, cannabidiolic acid (CBDA) has been found to be more effective than CBD at reducing nausea. Combining THC and CBDA with a patient's therapy may lead to better outcomes than THC and CBD alone.[158]

Studies have shown that when comparing cannabis and traditional medicine to placebo, a higher percentage of patients choose cannabis than choose traditional medicine. When comparing cannabis to traditional medication, the results are similar, with more people choosing cannabis over traditional medicine. However, when comparing the results of cannabis versus traditional medicine for the treatment of nausea/vomiting, the results are less clear. These studies show a higher incidence of adverse reactions in the cannabis groups, but these reactions may be beneficial in certain circumstances. Patients undergoing chemotherapy are often anxious and have difficulty sleeping. A euphoric sensation may help to alleviate anxiety, and drowsiness associated with cannabis use can promote sleep.[159] It could be these effects that guide patients into choosing cannabis over traditional medications.

Patient Reports S/S MS

Multiple Sclerosis is a degenerative disease of the nervous system that affects 2.5 million people worldwide. Patients that suffer from multiple sclerosis will suffer from spasticity (muscle spasms) as the disease progresses. These spasms can be painful and lead to other issues such as urinary and sleep disturbances, gait impairment, and mobility issues. These effects can lead to social isolation and depression, thus diminishing the quality of life of the patient, and lead to further negative effects such as skin breakdown and secondary infections. Over half of the patient's diagnosed with MS will report having symptoms of spasticity.[160]

The standard approach to MS spasticity is to treat the symptoms with a muscle relaxant. There is limited evidence that the most common medications—Zanaflex (tizanidine), Lioresal (baclofen), Valium (diazepam), and Dantrium (dantrolene)—are effective in this treatment.[161] All of these agents work to relax skeletal muscle which can in turn alleviate the spasticity associated with MS. If a patient is unresponsive to these medications, or is unable to tolerate them due to adverse effects, treatment options are limited.

Currently, there is only one cannabinoid product approved for use in MS. Sativex, a cannabinoid sublingual spray containing THC and CBD, is approved in the UK and several other countries including the EU, Canada, and Israel to treat spasticity resulting from MS. It achieves this effect by partially activating the CB1 and CB2 receptors located on the nerve terminals. By partially activating these receptors, the release of excitatory neurotransmitters is reduced and muscle stiffness is decreased leading to better muscle function. This is similar to the effect that our own endocannabinoids produce in the ECS.[162]

It has been shown that CBD can block the effects of MS and provide long term beneficial effects in mice studies.[163,164] When the disease is introduced to mice, CBD is able to provide protection to spinal tissue and facilitate repair to neurons that have been damaged. By improving this damage, symptoms are prevented and/or reduced. Researchers found that the mice treated with CBD after exposure had spinal cord tissue samples consistent to those that had not been exposed to the disease. One reason for this may be CBD's ability to increase the levels of BDNF, a growth factor, which in turn helps neurons heal after injury. Another possible explanation is that the anti-inflammatory response of CBD could inhibit the progression of neuronal damage from MS. Regardless, it was found that CBD helps to prevent the demyelination of neurons that leads to the symptoms and progression of MS.[165]

A study of 667 patients in the UK revealed a statistically significant reduction in muscle spasticity and pain as reported by MS patients. This study did not find a statistically significant reduction in muscle spasticity or pain as measured by the Ashworth Score (clinician measured response). This suggests a possible effect of cannabis altering the patient's perception of the muscle stiffness rather than improving the muscle stiffness itself.[166] Another study shows that patients reported a reduction in sleep disturbances from MS when using cannabis. The patients in this study similarly reported a reduction in pain and muscle spasticity when using cannabis.[167]

Weight Loss/Appetite Stimulation HIV/AIDS

One of the most common symptoms of HIV/AIDS is weight loss. The prevalence of this symptom is hard to point to due to changing definitions of wasting disease associated with HIV/AIDS. This is further complicated by researchers not knowing the exact mechanisms by which HIV/AIDS causes wasting syndrome. It is thought to be a multifaceted symptom caused by decreased appetite/caloric intake and changes in metabolism. Patients with HIV/AIDS can have decreased intake due to a variety of reasons such as nausea/vomiting, depression/anxiety, financial instability, or secondary infections. There can also be metabolic changes stemming from cytokine dysregulation and hormonal changes (such as hypogonadism) associated with the disease.[168]

There is no accepted standard for the treatment of wasting syndrome for HIV/AIDS. Treatment is tailored to the patient to achieve the best results. Treatment options include anabolic steroids, thalidomide, appetite stimulants, and Marinol (dronabinol).[169,170] Anabolic steroids (testosterone) can decrease patient weight loss by increasing muscle mass.[171] Steroids can be a good option in patients that are experiencing hypogonadism or low libido. Thalidomide is rarely used due to the potential for severe side effects, including birth defects.[172]

The appetite stimulants used for treating weight loss in HIV/AIDS encompass multiple drug categories. Megace (megestrol acetate) is FDA approved for HIV weight loss in HIV/AIDS patients. It is a synthetic derivative of progesterone, a hormone that the body naturally produces. While it has been shown to be effective in treating weight loss, its mechanism of action is unknown.[173] Remeron (mirtazapine) is a tetracyclic antidepressant. It has not been FDA approved for the treatment of weight loss in HIV/AIDS, but it has shown to be effective, as weight gain is one of its common side effects.[174]

Marinol (dronabinol) is the FDA approved synthetic version of THC. It has affinity for both CB1 and CB2 receptors but has a stronger effect on CB1 receptors. This promotes appetite stimulation, which in turn can decrease weight loss. In a placebo controlled study, THC was shown to improve appetite and maintain or increase body weight. Patients that continued dronabinol therapy in a secondary study after the end of the initial trial continued to see the benefits of improved appetite and weight gain.[175] This study found that even patients in the late stages of the disease had increased appetite and only modest weight loss.[176]

In the mid-1990s, it was shown that mice treated with THC experienced significant appetite stimulation over several hours with results returning to normal after 5-6 hours. At the time, the reason for this was unknown, but thought to be related to the brain's reward system and the way the mice's sensory receptors reacted to the food.[177] While the reward system may be a component in the success of cannabis inducing appetite stimulation, we now know that there is more involved. Later studies in mice proved that anandamide, 2-AG, and CB1 receptors were located in the hypothalamus. The hypothalamus controls the autonomic nervous system and feelings such as hunger and thirst. Mice that were given a dose of anandamide soon began overeating. The mice were then given a CB1 antagonist, and the overeating stopped. Other studies have shown that mice given a low dose of a CB1 agonist showed an increase in appetite while mice given high dose of the same CB1 agonist showed a decrease in appetite. In part, this is believed to be a result of increased stress and anxiety experienced by the mice at too high of a dose. These effects have been further supported by evidence from a study looking at newborn mice. Newborn mice that were given a dose of a CB1 antagonist stopped nursing. If the mice were then given a dose of THC, they resumed nursing again.[178]

Studies looking at cannabis for the treatment of appetite stimulation in humans uphold the results from mice studies. Dronabinol (FDA approved synthetic THC) has been associated with significant increased appetite above baseline, increased mood, and decreased nausea versus placebo. It was also noted that patients' weight was maintained while patients who were taking placebo lost weight.[179] In a study looking at weight loss in cancer patients, there was a significant decrease in the weight loss of cancer patients treated with dronabinol. Patients taking 2.5mg twice daily saw an almost 4 pound per month decrease in weight loss while patients taking 5mg twice daily saw a maintained weight or a slight weight gain.[180] In a double-blind, placebo-controlled cross-over study looking at THC versus placebo, it was found that patients taking THC exhibited a significant increase in appetite stimulating hormones.[181]

Tourette's

Tourette's syndrome (TS) is a neuropsychiatric disease that is characterized by involuntary tics. Tics are defined as sudden, rapid, recurrent, or nonrhythmic motor movements or vocalizations. Tics can range in severity from mild (blinking, throat clearing) to severe (shrugging, repeating last heard word). These tics are often socially disruptive and may appear to be exaggerated voluntary actions such as obscene gestures, imitating someone else's movements, or saying obscene, racist, or religious derogatory words. The tics can be associated with premonitory urges, and some patients are able to suppress them to varying degrees. For a diagnosis of TS, the tics must have persisted for more than one year, and the onset must be before the age of 18. The onset of tics is often seen in adolescence but peaks between the ages of 10 and 12. Males are between two to four times more likely to develop TS than females. TS is associated with other psychiatric disorders, with obsessive-compulsive disorder (OCD) and attention deficit hyperactivity disorder (ADHD) being common comorbidities.

Due to the complexity of TS and individual variations, there is no recommended guideline for the treatment of tics. For most patients (especially children), pharmacologic therapy is not indicated due to the severity of tics not interfering with the patient's daily life. Psychoeducation is often adequate treatment for these patients. Psychoeducation focuses on the symptoms of the disease and what can exacerbate them. It is often paired with behavioral therapy to increase its efficacy.

When a patient's tics begin to impair daily life, pharmacologic intervention may be necessary. The typical antipsychotics Haldol (haloperidol) and Orap (pimozide) have been shown to be effective in treating tics. Through double-blind studies, both have shown to be better than placebo, and haloperidol has shown to be more effective than pimozide. However, haloperidol has been shown to have more adverse reactions. While less studied, Prolixin (fluphenazine) has been shown to be effective and have fewer side effects than haloperidol.

Atypical antipsychotics also show benefit in treatment of tics. Risperdal (risperidone) has the highest level of evidence in this drug class. It has been found to have similar efficacy as haloperidol and pimozide. The benefit of risperdal is that it has fewer side effects compared to the typical antipsychotics.

Noradrenergic agents such as Catapres (clonidine), Tenex (guanfacine), and Strattera (atomoxetine) are generally used in children. These medications are primarily used for the treatment of ADD, so they may be of benefit in patients with comorbidities. Their effects are less than those of the antipsychotics and are used for mild to moderate tics.[182]

There is currently a limited amount of data available for the use of cannabis in the treatment of TS; however, what data we do have is promising. One small crossover designed, placebo controlled trial in humans has shown a significant reduction in motor tics (both simple and complex), reduction in simple vocal tics, and a decrease in obsessive-compulsive behaviors after treatment with THC as compared to placebo. These results are likely due to CB1 activation in the basal ganglia, an area of the brain associated with motor control, and the endocannabinoid systems interaction with the dopaminergic system.[183]

Another study looked at TS patients who were currently using cannabis to treat their symptoms. This study found that all participants self-reported clinically significant reduction in TS symptoms. The data shows a significant reduction in both motor and vocal tics. The researchers further broke down the data to reveal significant improvements in OCD and ADHD symptoms as well as decreases in irritability and anxiety.[184]

Generalized Anxiety Disorder

Generalized anxiety disorder (GAD) is defined as excessive anxiety and worry pertaining to multiple events or activities that the patient has trouble controlling or preventing from interfering with daily tasks. This anxiety is often associated with feeling on edge, being easily fatigued, concentration difficulties, irritability, muscle tension, and sleep disturbances. This excessive worrying impairs the patient's daily life. It can alter their ability to complete tasks efficiently at home or at work. GAD can also impair the patient's ability to get restful sleep by either preventing the patient from sleeping due to worrying thoughts or by causing restless, unsatisfying sleep. Typically, the onset of GAD happens around age 30, which is later in life than most other anxiety disorders; however, onset can develop early in some cases. Adults typically experience anxiety relating to day-to-day life issues such as finances, job stability, or daily tasks, whereas children experience anxiety focused on school or athletic performance. A big difference between GAD and normal anxiety is the patient's ability to manage the symptoms. In GAD, the symptoms are pervasive and controlling. With normal anxiety, a patient may be able to put off the anxiety if a more important or urgent matter comes up. Patients with GAD will often report additional symptoms such as trembling or feeling shaky, sweating, nausea, an exaggerated startle response, headaches, or irritable bowel syndrome. Unlike other anxiety disorders, symptoms such as increased heart rate, shortness of breath, and dizziness are not as commonly reported with GAD.[185]

Anxiety is generally treated with a selective serotonin reuptake inhibitor (SSRI), such as Prozac (fluoxetine) or Zoloft (sertraline), serotonin-norepinephrine reuptake inhibitor (SNRI), such as Cymbalta (duloxetine) or Effexor (venlafaxine), tricyclic antidepressant (TCA), such as Elavil (amitriptyline) or Pamelor (nortriptyline), or a benzodiazepine, such as Xanax (alprazolam) or Klonopin (clonazepam). Prescribers often choose an SSRI to initiate therapy as these drugs have the most evidence for effectiveness, the least amount of side effects, and are generally cost effective. TCA's are reserved for patients that are unable to tolerate an SSRI/SNRI or are unresponsive to treatment with these classes of medication. All three of these classes of drugs offer long term prevention of anxiety to patients, but they do require approximately four to six weeks of use before the effect is obtained. Benzodiazepines are used in patients that need a quick onset for anxiety relief, but these drugs do not provide long term prevention of anxiety. Benzodiazepines are often prescribed to patients to be used on an as-needed basis, either alone or in conjunction with an SSRI, SNRI, or TCA.[186] One major disadvantage with benzodiazepines is their interaction with opioid medications. Mixing a benzodiazepine and opioids can cause an increased risk of accidental opioid overdose leading to respiratory depression.[187]

In mice studies, it appears that CBD can be as effective as diazepam for the treatment of anxiety. Unlike diazepam which achieves its effect by activating benzodiazepine receptors, CBD achieves its effect through the activation of serotonin receptors. Another study shows that pretreating mice with CBD helps to mitigate both the flight response and the defensive immobility response when exposed to a predator. This is indicative of not only preventing anxiety but curbing anxiety attacks, another indication that serotonin receptors are being activated.[188] Further evidence of the serotonin receptor activation comes from the findings of CBD treated mice displaying reduced stress level of restraint, reduced anxiety related to repeated restraint, and the effect being reversed when given a serotonin antagonist in mice.[189]

THC is the active component of cannabis that is responsible for the psychoactive side-effects of the plant, including anxiety.[190] However, while high doses of THC can cause greater anxiety, it has been shown that low doses of THC can serve as an anxiolytic.[191] In human studies, the anxiolytic effect of CBD was first evidenced in the early 1980's during a study looking at the effects of cannabis in patients suffering from anxiety. In the study, participants were broken into multiple groups receiving either CBD, THC, THC plus CBD, diazepam, or a placebo. Anxiety was induced in the patients through a public speaking analogue, and each group received their respective treatment. It was found that patients that received CBD alone or the medication diazepam had significant reductions in anxiety levels. The researchers found that the group taking THC alone suffered higher anxiety levels than the group taking THC plus CBD.[192] This further suggests the role of CBD as an anxiolytic and highlights the benefit of a full spectrum product.

Human studies looking at anxiety rely on physical symptoms (increased heart rate, increased respiratory rate, sweating, etc.) as well as patient self-assessments to determine level of anxiety. There have been numerous studies looking at the effect of CBD since the original study using the methods mentioned above. One test in particular showed that patients receiving CBD had significantly lower levels of anxiety as measured by both physical symptoms and self-assessment survey results. While self-reporting is not the most scientifically reliable method for gauging treatment efficacy, both single photon emission computed tomography (SPECT) and functional magnetic resonance imaging (fMRI) have backed up these results by showing the positive effects of CBD on anxiety when examining brain activity in humans.[193]

Post-Traumatic Stress Disorder

Post-traumatic Stress Disorder (PTSD) is a psychiatric disorder experienced by people who have been exposed to traumatic events such as war, serious accidents, natural disasters, or violent assault. PTSD has been called various names throughout the years. During World War I and World War II it was referred to as "shell shock" and "combat fatigue", respectively. A traumatic event is defined as exposure to actual or threatened death, serious injury, or sexual violence. It is a common misconception that a person must experience combat to suffer from PTSD. While exposure to a traumatic event is necessary for the diagnosis of PTSD, it does not have to be a direct exposure. For instance, a person can develop PTSD from hearing about a close loved one's death. PTSD is characterized by intrusion symptoms (i.e., flashbacks), avoidance of stimuli that reminds the patient of the traumatic event, altered cognition and memories of the event, and altered reactivity (i.e., outbursts or exaggerated startle response). While symptoms of PTSD can occur months to years after the experience, it normally occurs within the first few months. PTSD is associated with social, occupational, and physical disabilities, high levels of medication usage, impaired social, interpersonal, and educational functions, as well as increased suicide risks. Patients with PTSD are 80% more likely to have a concurrent mental health disorder compared to those without PTSD.[194]

Patients with PTSD are often treated with selective serotonin reuptake inhibitors (SSRI) or serotonin-norepinephrine reuptake inhibitors (SNRI) such as Zoloft (sertraline), Paxil (paroxetine), Prozac (fluoxetine), and Effexor (venlafaxine) to combat the depression and anxiety associated with the disease. Medications in these drug classes are widely used to treat general depression and anxiety with varying results, and their effects are similar on PTSD patients. Prescription medication therapy is often used in conjunction with non-medication therapy to achieve the best results.[195,196]

A Canadian study has shown that nabilone (a synthetic cannabinoid that mimics THC) may be effective at treating nightmares associated with PTSD. While this study is small (10 patients), it is the first to look at the efficacy of a cannabinoid in treating symptoms of PTSD in a double-blind, placebo controlled study. Despite the small number of participants, researchers were able to determine statistical significance with the results. Seven, out of ten, participants saw significant improvement in their PTSD associated nightmares. This result is in line with other cohort studies that have been performed previously. [197]

94

Despite the promising results of this study, and studies currently under way, it is important for patients with PTSD to use caution when using medical cannabis. PTSD patients should only use medical cannabis under the supervision of a medical professional. Large, retrospective studies have conflicting answers on the benefits and dangers of cannabis and PTSD. There appears to be an association between cannabis use and severity of PTSD depression and suicidality.[198] One study shows an improvement in PTSD depression and suicidality after a four month break from using cannabis.[199] Because of the current conflicting data, and PTSD's association with substance abuse disorders, the use of medical cannabis for the treatment of PTSD will need to be evaluated on a case-by-case situation.

Glaucoma

Glaucoma is an ocular disease that can result in loss of vision or blindness resulting from damage to the optic nerve. This damage is caused by an increase in pressure in the eye. The eye contains a clear fluid that fills the front portion of the eye called the anterior chamber. This fluid is important for supplying the tissues of the eye with needed nutrients and is continuously flowing through the eye. However, when this fluid is not able to drain properly, pressure within the eye begins to increase. Any damage to the optic nerve from glaucoma cannot be reversed, so it is important that the disease is detected early and treatments are started promptly.

There are two major forms of glaucoma. Open angle glaucoma is characterized by a slowed draining of the fluid from the anterior chamber. Patients with open angle glaucoma will experience peripheral vision loss and, in severe cases, tunnel vision. This form of glaucoma is treated with eye drops intended to decrease fluid production or increase fluid drainage. Closed angle glaucoma occurs when fluid is unable to drain from the eye due to a blockage from the Iris. This constitutes a medical emergency and must be treated quickly, or blindness can occur. Symptoms of closed angle glaucoma include headache, nausea, red eye, and severe eye pain.[200]

The primary goal of therapy for glaucoma is to reduce intraocular pressure and to preserve vision. In the early stages of the disease, patients are typically treated through the use of prescription eye drops such as Xalatan (latanoprost) or Timoptic (timolol). These drops achieve their effect by allowing the aqueous humor to flow out of the eye and by reducing the production of aqueous humor, respectively.[201,202] Both of these mechanisms result in reduced intraocular pressure. Later stages of the disease, and closed angle glaucoma, may require surgical intervention.

Damage caused by glaucoma is two fold. First, increased ocular pressure leads to ischemic damage of the optic nerve. Second, increased levels of glutamate, likely caused by the increased pressure, cause cell death in the retinal ganglion cells.[203] Both THC and CBD have been shown to reduce the glutamate mediated cell death in glaucoma via antioxidant properties.[204] THC likely provides protection from activation of the CB1 receptors found in the retina.[205,206] CBD provides benefit by being both an antioxidant and by reducing the breakdown of anandamide. Anandamide is produced naturally by the endocannabinoid system and offers nueroprotevity to the retinal cells.[207]

A small, randomized, placebo-controlled study looked at the efficacy of THC and CBD at lowering intraocular pressure. This study found that two hours after giving sublingual THC, there was a significant lowering of intraocular pressure that returned to baseline four hours after dosing. While low dose CBD was shown to have no effect on lowering intraocular pressure, higher doses of CBD were found to increase intraocular pressure.[208]

Despite the lowering of intraocular pressure and glutamate levels, medical cannabis has the potential for exacerbating vision loss from damage to the optic nerve. This stems from cannabis' ability to lower blood pressure. By lowering blood pressure, the optic nerve could get less blood perfusion (blood flow through the tissues of the optic nerve). The lower perfusion can cause further damage to the already damaged optic nerve even after the intraocular pressure has been corrected. This risk has led the American Academy of Ophthalmology to urge caution to patients using medical cannabis to treat glaucoma.[209]

Hepatitis C

Hepatitis is defined as an inflammation of the liver. Hepatitis C (HCV) is a viral infection that is spread through contact with contaminated blood. It has two forms, acute and chronic. The acute form develops within months of exposure to the virus. Between 15-45% of people that develop acute HCV will not require treatment to overcome the virus. The 55-85% that are not able to overcome the virus will develop chronic HCV and require treatment. Around 75% of people with acute HCV do not experience any symptoms. Those that do may experience fatigue, nausea/vomiting, loss of appetite, gray colored stools, joint pain, or jaundice skin color. Those with chronic HCV generally do not develop symptoms until liver damage has occurred.

The standard therapy for treating HCV has been interferon-α (IFN-α) and ribavirin.[210] IFN-α elicits an increased immune response and suppresses cell proliferation through activation of specific enzymes.[211] While the mechanism of action for ribavirin is not completely understood, it is known to have antiviral effects and to inhibit the replication of HCV.[212] New understanding of the HCV disease process and clinical data supports using direct acting antivirals such as Harvoni (sofosbuvir/ledipasvir) to treat HCV.[213] Direct acting antivirals work by targeting proteins that are required for HCV to replicate and inhibiting the viral replication process.[214] These medications can cure HCV patients but come at a significant cost in the tens of thousands of dollars for treatment. It is estimated that a 12 week course of therapy for Harvoni would cost a patient nearly $95,000.[215]

In lab studies, CBD prevented replication of the HCV virus. In cells grown in the lab, CBD was nearly identical in effectiveness of virus inhibition as IFN-α (84.6% vs 85.4%).[216] However, these results have not been replicated in human trials. Human trials have shown that HCV patients using medical cannabis exhibit a statistically significant sustained viral response to treatment with interferon-α or ribavirin, decreased virologic relapse post-treatment, and increased medication adherence.[217] This is likely due to the ability of cannabis to treat the bothersome side effects of HCV medication therapy such as nausea/vomiting, loss of appetite, muscle pain, insomnia, and mood changes/disturbances.[218,219]

There is conflicting data on the safety of using medical cannabis in HCV patients. CB1 receptors have been located on stellate cells and myofibroblasts (two cell types that promote fibrosis). Mice that have been bred not to express CB1 receptors have shown reduced fibrosis in response to liver damage as opposed to normal mice. This effect was further confirmed when normal mice were given a CB1 antagonist and also showed reduced fibrosis in response to liver damage.[220] Alternatively, CB2 receptors are not found in normal, healthy liver cells. They are, however, found in cirrhotic liver cells caused by various disease states including HCV. These CB2 receptors were shown to decrease fibrosis by inhibiting fibral growth and by causing the cell death of fibrosis promoting cells. Further supporting this theory, mice that were bred to not express CB2 receptors were shown to have enhanced fibrosis in response to liver injury.[221] However, a greater incidence of moderate-to-severe fibrosis has been found in cannabis consumers than in non-cannabis users.[222] Because of these conflicting studies, it is important that HCV patients who want to use medical cannabis do so under the supervision of medical professionals until more studies can be performed to assess the safety and effectiveness of the treatment.

Amyotrophic Lateral Sclerosis

Amyotrophic Lateral Sclerosis (ALS), also known as Lou Gehrig's Disease, is a progressive neurodegenerative disease that affects both the upper and the lower motor neurons. As the disease progresses, it will eventually lead to the loss of muscle function. As this muscle function is lost, patients can lose the ability to move, walk, speak, eat, and eventually breath. Around 5-10% of people with ALS have the familial form of the disease. This means that they developed the disease through genes passed down from their parents. The offspring of a parent with ALS has around a 50% chance of developing the disease. The remaining 90% of people with the disease developed it randomly.[223]

Currently, there is only one FDA approved drug for the treatment of ALS. Rilutek (riluzole) has been approved by the FDA to prolong survival time and/or time to tracheotomy in patients with ALS. The exact mechanism by which it achieves this result is unknown, but one hypothesis is that by reducing glutamate release rates, it is able to protect motor neurons from inflammatory damage. This effect has been shown in both mice and human populations.[224]

In mice that have been genetically modified to develop an analogue for familial ALS, it has been shown through multiple studies that the ECS is both directly and indirectly involved with the development and progression of ALS.[225] These mice appear to have an increased sensitivity of CB1 receptor with regard to both inhibitory and excitatory synaptic transmission in the striatum and opposite rearrangements of glutamate and GABA mediated synaptic activity. These glutamate and GABA mediated activities govern the activity of the striatum.[226] Treatment of modified mice with a cannabinoid agonist significantly prevented progression of disease. By inhibiting fatty acid amide hydrolase (FAAH), which breaks down endogenous anandamide, the appearance of diseases signs were prevented. However, despite the signs of the disease being prevented, there was no improvement on lifespan. Ablating CB1 receptors has shown no effect on disease progression, but has extended lifespan. These results reinforce the idea of a neuroprotective role of cannabis and show a possible role of a non-CB1 receptor, possibly CB2, in the treatment of ALS.[227] This theory is further supported by the findings of increased CB2 receptors in the spinal tissue of patients with ALS.[228]

One of the major symptoms of ALS is pain. While there are currently no randomized, placebo-controlled studies looking at treating ALS pain with cannabis, we have previously discussed cannabis's ability to modulate pain.[229] There is substantial evidence to show that cannabis can reduce pain via its anti-inflammatory properties. It also appears that cannabis is able to directly modify the way the brain interprets pain signals. This two-fold effect could also explain the reason for patients reporting pain relief in ALS when treating with cannabis.

Other symptoms that cannabis can help control are excessive drooling, spasticity, appetite, and mood/anxiety. One of cannabis' more common side effects is dry mouth stemming from its ability to decrease saliva excretion. In patients with ALS, this side effect can serve a beneficial purpose. As mentioned in the MS section, patients report a significant decrease in spasticity when using cannabis. Cannabis has been reported to control ALS spasms in a similar nature. Cannabis' ability to stimulate appetite is one of its most known features. By stimulating appetite, it is possible cannabis could help to prevent decreased appetite leading to wasting syndrome in patients suffering from ALS. Lastly, cannabis has shown to lead to decreased anxiety levels and increased mood in patients. ALS patients often suffer from these symptoms and could find relief through medical cannabis treatment.[230]

Crohn's Disease and Ulcerative Colitis

Crohn's disease is an inflammatory bowel disease that can affect any part of the intestinal tract; however, it most commonly affects the small intestine and the beginning portion of the large intestine. The disease can start out slow and increase in severity over time. Some patients will experience periods of remission that can last up to years. Patients with Crohn's disease will experience diarrhea, painful abdominal cramping, and weight loss. It is unknown what the cause of Crohn's disease is, but researchers think it could be an autoimmune disorder or have a genetic component. Stress has been shown to increase the chance of Crohn's flare ups, but does not cause the disease to manifest itself.

Like Crohn's Disease, ulcerative colitis (UC) is an inflammatory bowel disease. The disease affects the inner lining of the large intestine and the rectum, and can cause sores or ulcers in these locations. Like

Crohn's, the disease starts off slow and can increase in severity over time. Patients can also have periods of remission that can last up to years with ulcerative colitis. Patients with UC will often experience painful diarrhea containing blood or purulent matter. Patients will also complain of an urgency to defecate but be unable to defecate.

Patients suffering from mild-to-moderate Crohn's disease may be treated with oral aminosalicylates such as Azulfidine (sulfasalazine) or a corticosteroid such as Entocort (budesonide). Moderate-to-severe patients may be treated with an oral corticosteroid, immunosuppressives such as Imuran (azathioprine) or Trexall (methotrexate), or anti-tumor necrosis factor agents such as Remicade (infliximab) or Humira (adalimumab).[231] Typically the anti-tumor necrosis factor agents (anti-TNF) are reserved for severe cases that are not responding well to other treatment. However, there is conflict over whether to start patients on an anti-TNF until remission is achieved and then step therapy down to maintain remission or continue the current process of starting with a corticosteroid and working up the list.[232]

Patients with mild-to-moderate UC typically receive an oral aminosalicylate, such as Azulfidine (sulfasalazine) or rectal mesalamine. Studies show that mesalamine has better outcomes, but some patients may delay starting due to the unpleasantness of using an enema or suppository. Patients that do not respond to these therapies may be given a corticosteroid such as prednisone in attempt to achieve remission. For patients that continue to to be unresponsive to treatment after corticosteroids, Imuran (azathioprine) may achieve the desired results. For severe cases that are unresponsive to these therapies, patients may be given Remicade (infliximab). [233]

Despite being different drug classes, the drugs mentioned in the previous paragraphs produce similar results. Aminosalicylates achieve their effect through anti-inflammatory and immunomodulatory mechanisms. They also achieve high concentration in the intestinal wall, making them a good choice for inflammatory bowel diseases.[234] Corticosteroids achieve their effect by reducing the inflammatory response of the diseases. Budesonide has a strong anti-inflammatory effect when used topically. Since Crohn's disease affects the intestinal tract, this effect is obtained by using time release capsules that do not dissolve until they reach the intestinal tract. The medicine is absorbed into the bloodstream, and then metabolized by the liver, thus limiting systemic side effects.[235] Immunosuppressives reduce inflammation in the way that their name suggests. By modulating the immune response, the body does not react as strongly to the disease and thus creates less inflammation around the affected tissues.[236] Patients with inflammatory bowel diseases have been found to have increased levels of TNF-α. Anti-TNF factor medication works by blocking TNF-α from binding with its receptor. When activated, this receptor releases inflammatory mediators eliciting an inflammatory response.[237,238]

While these two disease states (UC and Crohn's disease) are different, their treatment with cannabis is similar. Animal studies have shown that activating CB1 receptors leads to decreased intestinal motility and reduced GI transit time.[239] We know that humans have used cannabis since ancient times to treat disorders of the intestines. It hasn't been until recent history, though, that we discovered that the lining of the intestinal wall and the enteric nervous system (ENS), the part of the nervous system that controls the contractility, and thus motility, of the intestines, contains CB receptors.[240] It has been found that activating CB receptors in the enteric nervous system and in the epithelial lining of the intestine leads to a decrease in acetylcholine release resulting in decreased intestinal contractility and peristalsis.[241]

Tissue samples have shown that in patients with UC, there is a decrease in the level of anandamide produced by the endocannabinoid system; however, there is an increase in the expression of CB2 receptors in the intestinal tract. This is likely due to the increased inflammation stemming from the disease state.[242] Activation of these receptors could lead to lessening of symptoms due to CB2 receptor anti-inflammatory effect.

CB1 receptors in the ENS serve as a way to decrease the overstimulation caused by IBS.[243] Excessive stimulation of the ENS causes hypermotility leading to diarrhea. Decreasing this stimulation will lead to lessened cramping and diarrhea. There is the possibility of a central CB receptor effect as well. Activation of CB1 and CB2 receptors in the brain can account for the decreased pain and nausea that UC and Crohn's patients report experiencing.[244]

In a study comparing sulfasalazine (a common medication for treating ulcerative colitis and Crohn's disease) to THC alone, CBD alone, or THC/CBD combo in mice, it was found that all three reduced inflammation, damage to intestinal lining, and functional disturbances. While all three medications showed positive benefits, THC showed the best outcomes as it improved symptoms of the disease as well as protected the cholinergic neurons from further damage. Furthermore, it was found that a THC/CBD combination with a less than effective dose of THC (when compared to THC alone) did have therapeutic effect, highlighting the entourage effect of cannabis products.[245]

Alzheimer's Disease

Alzheimer's disease is a brain disorder that affects the memory and thinking skills of sufferers. The damage caused by the disease is progressive and irreversible. The disease can start out mild with little effect on the patient's daily life. As the disease progresses, it will cause the patient to develop behavioral and psychological effects. These effects can be more disturbing to the patient than the cognitive effects, especially in the early stages. These effects are often what push the patient to seek help from their medical provider. For late stage patients, agitation, combativeness, wandering, gait disturbances, incontinence, and seizures are common.

Ultimately, the disease results in death. The disease can progress at different rates. The mean survival after diagnosis is 10 years, but this is not necessarily due to the disease itself. The disease often presents in elderly patients that have multiple health conditions. Patients that are diagnosed earlier in life will often progress through the entire disease and can live up to 20 years or possibly more post-diagnosis.[246] While the typical age of onset for Alzheimer's is in the mid-60s, the damage that leads to memory loss and function can begin decades earlier. In patients with the disease, abnormal protein deposits form amyloid plaques that disrupt neuron paths, leading to the neurons dying. This process starts in the hippocampus region of the brain (the region responsible for memory formation) and spreads to other regions as it progresses. As each region is affected, the neurons located in that region begin to die, resulting in shrinkage. By late stage Alzheimer's, the brain has shrunk significantly due to this process.

There are currently two classes of medication that have FDA approval for the treatment of Alzheimer's, acetylcholinesterase inhibitors, such as Exelon (rivastigmine) or Aricept (donepezil), prescribed for patients with mild-moderate Alzheimer's and NMDA antagonists, Namenda (memantine), prescribed for patients with moderate-severe Alzheimer's.[247] Acetylcholinesterase inhibitors work by increasing the levels of acetylcholine in the brain by blocking its breakdown by the enzyme acetylcholinesterase. Increased acetylcholine leads to increased cholinergic function. This increased cholinergic function can improve some of the cognitive effects of the disease. While improving symptoms, this class of medication does not reverse or stop the progression of the disease.[248] NMDA antagonists work by inhibiting the neurotransmitter glutamate. Increased levels of glutamate leads to increased excitotoxicity and, ultimately, neuronal damage. By decreasing the glutamate levels, some of the symptoms of Alzheimer's are alleviated. Like the acetylcholinesterase inhibitors, NMDA antagonists reverse or stop the progression of Alzheimer's.[249]

It is thought that B-amyloid peptide aggregates play a part in the destructive process of Alzheimer's by inducing oxidative stress. This has been shown in rats that were injected with B-amyloid peptide. These rats showed signs of increased reactive oxygen species, and caspase 3 (an enzyme associated with cell death) was detected. However, in rats treated with CBD prior to being given B-amyloid peptide, cell survival was increased via a reduction in reactive oxygen species, and caspase 3 levels were lower. This suggests that CBD has neuroprotective, antioxidant, and cell saving properties.[250] Further studies in mice show that a decreased expression of CB1 receptors can lead to worsened Alzheimer's-related cognitive effects.[251]

There have been limited trials looking at the use of cannabinoids for treatment of Alzheimer's in humans. While these studies are limited due to small patient size, they do give insight into how cannabis affects Alzheimer's in the human population. Looking at post-mortem human tissue samples yields conflicting results in regards to CB1 regulation in Alzheimer's patients. Some studies show a decreased level of CB1 expression while others show no change. However, there is a significant increase in CB2 expression in Alzheimer's patients. These increased levels are associated with the pathological changes from the disease but not with the cognitive changes.[252] Most studies evaluating the efficacy of THC in Alzheimer's have been performed with dronabinol (FDA approved synthetic THC). Dronabinol has been found to increase body weight, decrease severity of disturbing behavior, and decrease nocturnal motor activity and agitation in severely demented patients.[253,254] The ECS, specifically CB1 receptors, has been shown to cause vasodilation leading to increased cerebral blood flow.[255] This could be of benefit to Alzheimer's patients by increasing oxygen and nutrient flow to the affected parts of the brain. Lastly, as discussed in previous sections, cannabinoids play a role in alleviating depression and anxiety. These same effects can be of benefit to patients suffering from Alzheimer's.

Epilepsy

There are 3.4 million people living in the United States with epilepsy with an estimated 150,000 new cases each year.[256] Epilepsy is the condition of having recurrent seizures, or interruptions in normal cell signaling in the brain leading to interruption of normal brain function. Because of this broad definition, the term "epilepsy" applies to more than one type of seizure.[257] These seizures can stem from numerous causes including brain injury from trauma or cerebrovascular event, infection, birth defect, hereditary trait, or

105

any other cause of brain injury.[258] The minimum requirement for diagnosing epilepsy is experiencing one unprovoked epileptic seizure and a brain abnormality that increases the chances of experiencing another. Without findings of an abnormality, the diagnosis requires two unprovoked epileptic seizures.[259]

Epileptic seizures can have a focal onset (one area of the brain, previously called partial-onset), generalized onset (both sides of the brain), or an unknown onset. Determining the onset location can be challenging for medical staff. Focal onset seizures can be mistaken for generalized onset seizures due to the complex propagation routes the seizures follow. Generalized onset seizures can affect one side of the body thus appearing to be focal onset. Unknown onset seizures are typically the result of a seizure occurring when the patient is asleep or alone and cannot remember the details of the seizure. However, not all seizure sufferers will lose awareness. Depending on the location of the seizure in the brain, some patients will remember the details from the event and can help medical staff classify the type of seizure.[260]

Patients newly diagnosed with focal point seizures may be treated with a variety of medications, either solo or in combination. Medicines with the most evidence for effectiveness include Tegretol (carbamazepine), Dilantin (phenytoin), Mysoline (primidone), Depakote (divalproic acid), or Sabril (vigabatrin). As with focal point seizures, patients with generalized onset seizures may be treated with a variety of medications. Many of the available choices are the same medications used to treat focal point seizures while some are different. Medications with the most evidence for effectiveness include Tegretol (carbamazepine), Neurontin (gabapentin), Trileptal (oxcarbazepine), Dilantin (phenytoin), Lamictal (lamotrigine), Topamax (topiramate), or Depakote (divalproic acid).[261] Despite these medications being from multiple drug classes, and having multiple mechanisms of action, they are able to treat multiple seizure types by blocking the seizure propagation through the inhibition of neuronal excitation.[262,263,264,265,266,267,268,269,270]

106

The first recorded use of cannabis for the treatment of seizures is from 1843 in which a 40-day old infant having recurrent seizures was given a cannabis tincture, and the seizures subsided. Interestingly, it was documented that after the initial dosing, the tincture was stored improperly, unbeknownst to the doctor. The doctor details that when the seizures returned, the tincture did not work as it did the first time. Upon discovery of the improper storage, it was determined the infant only received water drops as the alcohol had evaporated and the cannabis resin stuck to the sides of the vial. Once the tincture was remade, the seizures were once again brought under control.[271]

The ECS has been found in areas of the brain affected by epilepsy. Specifically, CB1 receptors have been found in the hippocampus and cerebellum, among others sites. In patients suffering from epilepsy, the expression of these receptors are increased.[272] THC is the most widely studied cannabinoid in epilepsy. It does appear to have some antiepileptic effect through its interaction with CB1 receptors in the brain, but there are studies showing exacerbation of seizures. This fact, along with its psychoactive side effects, has led researchers to focus on CBD and cannabidivarin (CBDV) for the treatment of epilepsy. In studies looking at induced seizures in mice and rats, CBD has shown anti-seizure properties in multiple seizure types, including epilepsy. The mechanism of action for this is still unknown as CBD has a weak affinity for CB1 receptors, but it is thought that non-CB receptors are being activated to achieve this result. CBDV has also shown to be effective in treating epileptic seizures in rats while maintaining no psychoactive effect.[273]

In 2018, the FDA approved Epidiolex (cannabidiol) for the treatment of Lennox-Gastaut syndrome and Dravet syndrome in patients 2 years of age and older. Epidiolex is the first product approved by the FDA that is derived from a cannabis plant rather than being synthesized in a lab. Two randomized, placebo controlled trials looking at Lennox-Gastaut syndrome showed a greater reduction in seizures in patients taking Epidiolex versus placebo. One study looking at Dravet syndrome showed a significant reduction in seizures in patient taking Epidiolex versus placebo with 6.7% of patients taking Epidiolex having no seizures versus 0% of placebo patients reporting no seizures.[274] The approval of Epidiolex has set up a confusing legal status for CBD. Epidiolex, plant derived CBD, is considered a schedule V medication by the DEA; however, plant derived CBD that is not from GW Pharmaceuticals under the name of Epidiolex is still considered schedule I and illegal by the DEA unless the CBD was derived from a producer under the regulations of a state sanctioned industrial hemp pilot research program.[275] We will touch on the legality of CBD later in this primer. Despite Epidiolex's narrow treatment indication and significant cost ($32,500 a year), the drug gives patients a clearly legal avenue to access CBD. Insurance coverage and potential off-label prescribing may increase legal access to CBD for a more significant population of patients.

Chapter 12: Types of Cannabis Medicine

Inhalable

Flower

The quality of dried and cured flowers of the cannabis plant are sorted into three tiers. The first tier is the best quality product that is displayed on the sales floor and sold by weight. The second tier is essentially as efficacious as the first tier, but is aesthetically inferior in some way (typically less dense bud structure or leafier, also called "larfy"). This second tier can be either processed into pre-rolled joints or sold at a discounted rate. The third tier is what is commonly called "shake" or "trim." "Shake" is the small pieces that fall off the cannabis bud as a result of regular handling. "Trim" is the pieces that are removed from the cannabis plant before it is cured. The third tier is generally sold at discounted rates in pre-rolled joints or in bulk. Many people turn this third tier into extracts in order to optimize the phytochemical content.

Concentrates and Extracts

There are a multitude of processes through which compounds can be retrieved from cannabis. Extracts are concentrates that have been made using a solvent (all extracts are concentrates, but not all concentrates are extracts). The process used will affect the compounds more likely to be present, but ultimately end product potency testing is most reliable to determine phytochemical profile of the specific medicine. Except for tinctures and oil infusions, the solvents used for extraction should not be found in the end product. Concentrates range from including complete plant material to isolating pure phytochemicals. If the process includes applying heat, the cannabinoids will become decarboxylated (converting the acid form of the phytochemical to a neutral form). Decarboxylated and non-decarboxylated cannabinoids can have different effects on the body. Degradation of phytochemicals can occur due to heat, humidity, light, oxygen, acid, and enzymes. Degradation is not always perceived as a negative event. When THC is oxidized it converts to CBN. CBN is known to have increased sedative properties, so it may be an appealing cannabinoid for treating insomnia.

Terminology varies in the cannabis community, but common conceptual terms are:

- Concentrates
  - *Kief*: powder-like substance (usually collected by sifting plant material through a screen) resulting from trichomes separating from bud and leaf plant material.
  - *Hash*: compressed kief.
  - *Rosin*: heated and compressed bud and leaf plant material (rather than just the kief).

Kief, hash and rosin are usually consumed via combustion inhalation or vaporization inhalation.

- Concentrate Extracts
  - *Tincture*: dried plant material placed in a solvent that can be safely consumed (alcohol or glycerine are examples). After a period of time, the plant material is strained and the resulting extract can be orally consumed as-is, or diluted for consumption.
  - *Oils*
    - Oil extraction via infusion: dried plant material placed in a consumable oil, usually heated, strained and orally consumed as-is, diluted for consumption, or added to other ingredients for edibles or topicals.
    - Oil extraction via solvent whereby the solvent is removed: plant material is processed using solvents (such as CO_2, alcohol, ethanol, and butane), heat and/or pressure separate phytochemicals from the solvent, and the separated phytochemicals result in an oil. Additional extraction methods can further separate subsequent phytochemicals out of the oil.

Phytochemical content and process techniques impact the viscosity level of the oil.

- *Full extract cannabis oil* [FECO] or full extract hemp oil [FEHO] contains more plant compounds including cannabinoids, terpenes, flavonoids, chlorophyll and plant lipids. Full extract oil is usually orally consumed or added to topicals.

- *Full spectrum cannabis oil*: contains an array of (at least) cannabinoids and terpenes, but the chlorophyll and some lipids have been removed. Full spectrum oil can be orally consumed as-is, diluted for consumption, or added to other ingredients for edibles or topicals. Certain CO_2 oils can be inhaled via vaporization. While some products use other types of processed full spectrum oil for vape cartridges (usually cut with polyethylene glycol, propylene glycol, vegetable glycerine, or medium chain triglycerides) the lipids left in the oil and the additive ingredients make it a less desirable vaporized medicine compared to distillate with terpenes added back in.

- *Distillate*: contains mostly cannabinoids and some lipids. Chlorophyll, some lipids, and terpenes are removed in the process. Some distillate has terpenes reintroduced to enhance aroma and flavor. Distillate can be orally consumed as-is, diluted for consumption, added to other ingredients for edibles or topicals, and inhaled via vaporization or combustion.

  - Additional consistencies in concentrate extracts exist beyond oil. These extracts are predominantly made using butane. Examples are:
    - Shatter
    - Snap and Pull
    - Wax

111

○ *Crystalline*, also known as *isolate*: results from multiple extraction and distillation methods that result in isolated cannabinoid crystals. Isolate can also take a powder form. Isolate can be suspended for consumption, added to other ingredients for edibles or topicals, and inhaled via vaporization.

Edible

Cannabis can be combined with almost any food item, given that a few core principles are followed in their creation. Heat can be applied directly to the cannabis flower which can then be used as the base material in an edible or capsule, or one of the extraction processes can be utilized wherein heat is applied and the end extract is ready for oral consumption as is. Often, the extracts are created with food grade oils or emulsified into them to increase their efficacy. This is because cannabinoids bind to fat molecules, and binding them to healthy Omega 3's (like coconut oil) helps them pass the blood/brain barrier.

Topical

Cannabis topicals can be prepared as lotions, salves, balms, chapsticks, bath salts, roll-on oils, and rubs, among other preparations. Each of these preparations will have a different level of therapeutic effect based on the absorption rate of the base, potency of cannabinoids, and application method used. Note that some mild psychoactive effect can be achieved if a permeable membrane interacts with the topical solution, such as when soaking in bath salts.

Permeables

Transdermal patches are a relatively new delivery method in cannabis medicine. Transdermal patches are applied topically to the skin to allow the medication to be absorbed in a time-release fashion (typically over a 24 hour period). Transdermal patches offer a more consistent effect than edible forms of medical marijuana. This is due to the release rate being controlled by the patch itself and not the body's metabolism. They require specialized equipment to produce, tend to be more expensive than equivalent options, and are prone to irritation when removed, but can provide stable, long-term relief when alternate forms of consumption are insufficient.

Chapter 13: Methods of Consumption

Inhaling

The most common method of cannabis consumption is through inhalation. Inhaling cannabis provides the most immediate effect and the shortest duration of action. Inhalation can involve smoking, vaporizing, or nebulizing cannabis products such as dried or cured flowers or concentrated cannabis oil extract. Vape pens allow for a more metered dose by using vaporizer cartridges and a heating element that is powered by a mobile battery. Studies investigating the potential connection between cannabis inhalation and cancers of the pulmonary system have shown no correlation between the two. For patients with coexisting respiratory conditions, however, additional irritation of the lungs should be avoided.

Oral

Consuming cannabis orally has more potent effect but a longer onset of action due to a different metabolic route through the liver that produces 11-hydroxy THC. The liver can be bypassed by using a tincture form of cannabis. The tincture is absorbed through the buccal membrane, resulting in an effect similar to inhalation methods. Products such as medicated lozenges will utilize both pathways as some of the medication being used sublingually is also swallowed. Keep in mind that your body will absorb the contents of a liquid faster than a solid edible such as a brownie. As such, you will experience the effects sooner (45 minutes vs 1-2 hours), the peak effect will be more intense, and the effect will dissipate quicker (4 - 8 hours). The use of raw or heated cannabis produces varied effects when creating edible cannabis products. Heating cannabis (decarboxylation) converts the acid forms of the cannabinoids into the more biologically active metabolites.

Topical

The topical application of cannabinoid compounds can provide localized relief without psychoactive effects due to the cannabinoid receptors found in the skin. As with more traditional methods, individual cannabinoids will interact with the receptors differently, resulting in varied therapeutic effects. When combined with other phytochemicals, cannabinoid compounds can be used in pain relief, reduced muscle inflammation/tenderness, decreased swelling, mitigated skin damage, and even alleviated migraine symptoms. Extracts and infused oil can be applied directly to the skin, but they are typically combined with other compounds to increase efficacy. Cannabinoids can be included in lotions, bath salts, balms, oils, and sprays.

Other

There are several additional routes of administration that are possible but are not as prevalent. Anal suppositories are considered by some to be the most medically efficacious delivery mechanism, as it delivers cannabinoids directly to the bloodstream without being metabolized by the liver. Vaginal suppositories are gaining popularity in the treatment of severe menstrual symptoms. Transdermal delivery systems also deliver cannabinoids directly to the bloodstream but can cause irritation to the areas where the patch is applied. Some of the newest medical cannabis formulations available include intranasal delivery, metered dose inhalers, and nebulizers.

Chapter 14: Dosage

To minimize adverse side effects and potential harmful drug interactions, it is important for the team of patient, physician and pharmacist to be mindful about benefit-risk analysis. Studies have shown that slower titration at lower doses have a marked reduction in adverse events while also improving the therapeutic efficacy of the medical cannabis.[276] A "low and slow" dosing protocol, starting with low THC and higher CBD content and utilizing quarterly cannabis detoxes, is the most appropriate protocol for most medical cannabis patients.

While it is nearly impossible to fatally overdose from consuming cannabis, it is possible for one's faculties to be altered to the point of physical and/or psychological discomfort. In order to appreciate cannabis for its health and healing properties, ensure safe consumption practices, and support (rather than further imbalance) the endocannabinoid system towards homeostasis, patients should use a low and slow medicating protocol. Patients consuming cannabis for the first few times should:

- Be at home or in a comfortable, private setting
- Choose a time to consume that would allow rest/sleep if they become tired or if they experienced unpleasant side effects
- Limit persons around to only those that are aware the patient is consuming cannabis as a new user, are supportive of the process, and that the patient feels very comfortable being around
- Have a glass of water nearby for quenching thirst or aiding with dry-mouth side effects (adding fresh ginger, lemon or lime, and/or mint can also be helpful)
- Prepare some healthy snacks or meals before hand, in case they become hungry

When starting cannabis medicine for the first time, it is recommended to use an inhaled consumption method unless the condition does not allow for inhalation of cannabis medicine. If the patient cannot initiate consumption of cannabis via inhalation, they should begin with oral consumption.

117

Inhaling Cannabis Medicine

A patient should start with a low-to-no-THC:CBD ratio smokable flower (using a glass piece designed for low-to-moderate consumption, such as a one-hitter, and using a hemp/beeswax wick to light the flower in place of a match or lighter) or vaporizable flower or concentrate (using a vaporization delivery mechanism designed for low-to-moderate consumption, such as an adjustable Volcano, Quill, or Pax). Using a natural breath pattern, they should inhale one to three times with three minutes between each individual inhalation. It is not preferable to hold in the cannabis medicine—rather to breath in-and-out naturally.

The feelings derived from inhaled consumption of cannabis usually peak between fifteen to thirty minutes and conclude after two to three hours. The conservative low and slow dosing protocol should be maintained every three to four hours for three to five days. The amount consumed per dose can be increased after three to five days in increments of one to three inhalations and/or one to three times the depth of breath (while still not holding the cannabis in – always inhaling and exhaling in a fluid motion). The potency can be increased, and/or the phytochemical profile changed, after a nine to fifteen day cycle of dosing. If the patient experiences adverse effects that are unmanageable or imbalanced in relation to the relief, they should discontinue use immediately and consult a medical or cannabis professional to adjust the potency and/or phytochemical profile of the medicine.

Once inhaled cannabis medicine has been introduced to the body and a patient feels comfortable with its effects, they may want to, or it may be advantageous to, introduce oral consumption of cannabis medicine. Oral consumption can replace or work in tandem with inhaled consumption; however, it is best for a patient to begin oral consumption protocol without the effects of inhaled cannabis consumption still evident in the body (best after a full night of sleep).

Oral consumption

Medicinal products designed for oral consumption are usually made from one of three base processes: tincture, infused oil, or extracted/concentrated oil. The low and slow protocol should be followed in that order: tincture, infused oil, then extracted/concentrated oil. No matter the type of edible, similar to inhalation, it is best to begin with a low-to-no-THC:CBD ratio product at or below five milligrams per dose.

Tinctures

Tinctures are the first edible product in the low and slow protocol because they affect the body in a similar fashion as inhalation. A patient should consume the number of drops of tincture that equates to one milligram, wait three minutes between each one milligram dose, and not exceed five milligrams. The feelings derived from tincture consumption of cannabis usually peak between fifteen to thirty minutes and conclude after two to three hours. The conservative low and slow dosing protocol should be maintained every three to four hours for three to five days. The amount consumed per dose can be increased after three to five days in increments of one to five milligrams. The potency, and/or change in phytochemical profile, of the dose can be increased after a nine to fifteen day cycle of dosing. If adverse effects that are unmanageable or imbalanced in relation to the relief are experienced, use should be discontinued immediately, and a pharmacist should be consulted to adjust the potency and/or phytochemical profile of the medicine.

Oil/Extract/Concentrates

Cannabis infused oil and cannabis extract/concentrate oil behave differently in the body compared to inhalation and tinctures. They can have heightened effects, delayed onset, and last longer. Similar to tinctures, they should be consumed at or below a five milligram dose. Onset may take one to three hours, peak in the range of two to five hours, and have a duration time of five to ten hours. Patients should start at one dose at or below five milligrams every six to eight hours for three to five days before decreasing the time between doses or the dosage amount. The potency, and/or change in phytochemical profile, of dose can increase after a nine to fifteen day cycle of dosing. If adverse effects that are unmanageable or imbalanced in relation to the relief are experienced, a patient should discontinue use immediately and consult a medical or cannabis professional to adjust the potency and/or phytochemical profile of the medicine.

Additional Considerations

Patients should refrain from driving or operating heavy machinery for at least three hours after consuming inhaled cannabis or at least eight hours after consuming cannabis orally. Patients should be mindful that cannabis can increase the effects of prescribed opiate painkillers and pharmaceuticals that may cause drowsiness. Cannabis may act synergistically with alcohol (increasing the effects of the cannabis and alcohol), so alcohol should not be consumed for at least three hours after consuming inhaled cannabis or eight hours after consuming cannabis orally. Cannabis should not be used while still under the effects of alcohol. Patients should consult a medical or cannabis professional for additional guidance regarding other prescription drug interactions and cannabis medicine.

Chapter 15: Adverse Effects

Cannabis, like any other medication, can have adverse effects and drug interactions. These effects can range from mild (dry mouth, increased appetite) to severe (heart palpitations, platelet inhibition). As such, patients should perform a risk-to-benefit analysis with their primary health care provider and/or pharmacist to ensure that cannabis is the right choice for them.

Discussing side effects of medical cannabis requires nuance, because what is negatively perceived for one condition may be seen as beneficial for another. For example, the over-the-counter medication diphenhydramine (Benadryl) is used to treat allergy symptoms (runny nose, sneezing, watery eyes, etc.), but when taken, it causes the patient to become drowsy. This is a side-effect of taking the diphenhydramine. However, if a patient takes an over-the-counter sleep aid product, it likely contains diphenhydramine as the active ingredient. In this case the drowsiness is the *intended* effect, not a side-effect.

Acute Effects

The varied phytochemical makeup of a specific formulation can also alter the perceived effect. Potential adverse effects of cannabis have been described in several reports.[277,278,279] Common side effects include the following:

- Dry mouth (often referred to as "cottonmouth")
- Dry and/or red eyes
- Increased appetite (often referred to as the "munchies")
- Unexpected increase in unfocused energy
- Increased sedation or lethargy

The same appetite, energy, and sleep effects can be beneficial depending on condition symptom relief desired. If a patient is suffering from insomnia, the CNS depressive effects of cannabis can induce sleep. If a patient has been diagnosed with cachexia, the appetite stimulation becomes a beneficial effect. These side effects tend to resolve within one to four hours.

Increased dosage amount and/or concentration can produce varied effects. For example, the same medical cannabis product at a low level can have anxiolytic effects while at a high level can increase or amplify anxiety. Acute adverse side effects attributed to consuming too much cannabis (overdose) include:

- Panic
- Paranoia
- Hallucinations
- Heart palpitations
- Shortness of breath
- Nausea
- Cold sweats
- Shaking or trembling
- Extreme lethargy/sedation resulting in immobilization

These effects are more commonly seen in high THC medical cannabis products compared to low-to-no THC products. By using the entourage effect and limiting phytochemical isolation, these adverse effects can be mitigated.

If acute adverse effects are experienced by a patient, there are steps that can be taken to alleviate the symptoms. Advise patients to remain calm; the feelings will pass, usually within twelve hours. Recommend a relaxing activity to take the patient's mind off the feelings of discomfort. Drinking plenty of fluids and eating a healthy snack such as whole fruit will increase possible low blood sugar. As with any medication that causes CNS depression, recommend the patient refrain from driving or operating heavy machinery while under the influence. CBD can alleviate some of the physiological effects associated with cannabis toxicity,[280] though it does not reduce the psychotropic feeling of being high.[281] A low THC:CBD ratio is commonly recommended to new patients in order to minimize psychological discomfort and maximize therapeutic effect.

These effects can be very uncomfortable, but it is important to note cannabis alone cannot cause a fatal overdose.[282] Endocannabinoid receptors are not found in abundance in the parts of the brain that support vital functioning such as respiration and circulation. Most illicit drugs that cause fatal overdoses affect these areas. Pharmaceutical medications that cause fatal overdoses affect these areas, or can be combinations of drugs that can include acetaminophen (as an example), which, taken in excess, can cause liver failure. Cannabis has shown to be both non-lethal and non-toxic. The adverse effects from cannabis overdose will subside usually within 2-12 hours.

Long-term Effects

Longitudinal studies of chronic adverse effects are not prevalent and have resulted in a variety of opposing conclusions.[283] No long-term negative side effects are currently associated with intermittent or low-to-moderate cannabis use. In general, there are concerns about long-term effects on brain development and memory in adolescents who are heavy cannabis users. Adults who are heavy cannabis users seem to have higher chances of developing anomic aphasia, or a problem with word recall. Regular users of inhaled cannabis have a higher risk of chronic bronchitis and impaired respiratory function. Cannabis' relationship to heart conditions may very well not be causal, but rather correlate to enhancing cardiovascular issues related to an existing condition.[284] Because of inadequate data, women should avoid consuming cannabis while pregnant and breastfeeding.

Long-term concerns regarding cannabis addiction, mental health, and social functioning seem to be intertwined. Longitudinal studies point to predisposition toward mental health conditions and social positioning as correlative with cannabis use as it relates to long-term mental health concerns, education attainment, and self-sufficiency.[285] Patients with pre-existing mental health conditions and their health care providers should be mindful of the benefit-to-risk analysis of medical cannabis use when determining the best treatment strategies.

Statistically, cannabis has a 6-10% addiction rate.[286] This is a lower addiction rate than tobacco, alcohol, and some prescription drugs, but nonetheless should be a consideration when evaluating the appropriateness of therapy for individual patients.

Chapter 16: Drug Interactions

As with any other medication, drug interactions should be checked before a patient starts a medical cannabis regimen. Owing to the need for more research, the fundamental ambiguity of the endocannabinoid system, and the wide range of pharmacologically active compounds potentially present in any cannabis formulation, it is very difficult to definitively list drug interactions. It is important to note that there are numerous pertinent compounds in cannabis, and they need to be specifically examined for how they interact with other pharmaceuticals.

Cannabis is suspected to decrease platelet aggregation,[287] induce CYP2E1, inhibit CYP3A4 and P-glycoprotein, and function as a CNS depressant. Patients should be cautious using cannabis while they are taking CNS depressants, anticholinergics, or sympathomimetics due to potential increased chances of side effects.[288] THC is metabolised by CYP2C9 and CYP3A4, while CBD is metabolized by CYP2C19 and CYP3A4. Medications which inhibit these enzymes can increase the plasma concentrations of THC and CBD, leading to adverse effects. Conversely, a potent inducer of these enzymes can render the cannabis dose ineffective. There is the potential for cannabis to cause hypomanic events in patients who are taking disulfiram or fluoxetine. The evidence for this interaction comes from the Marinol® drug trials in which two case reports (one for each medication) detailed this adverse effect. While it may not be of importance to most patients on these medications, special care should be used in patients that suffer from bipolar disorder or are prone to manic events. Modification of prescription dosages may need to be considered through assessment of the effects of the medical cannabis.

Case reports are useful in calling attention to the extreme potentials of a drug and can spur more robust research into important topics like pharmacodynamic interactions. This research can be as rudimentary as aggregating these case reports and analyzing the group data. There are myriad individual case reports that are often pointed to as being definitive statements on the dangers of drug interactions with cannabis, such as one detailing the case of a 17 year old male who was taking amitriptyline 25mg at bedtime for sleep and depression. Shortly after starting the medication, he was admitted to the ER and diagnosed with supraventricular tachycardia with a rate of 300 bpm. The teen admitted to smoking cannabis the day before, and a search of his home, and interviewing of his friends, turned up no other drug or alcohol use. The ER physician attempted to convert to normal sinus rhythm with an IV dose of verapamil, but ultimately the patient had to be transferred to the ICU for electroconversion.[289]

Another case report shows the case of a 56 year old male being treated with warfarin while using cannabis to treat depression. He was admitted to the hospital for an upper GI bleed, and it was discovered his INR was 10.41 with a hemoglobin of 6.6 g/dL. The next day his INR was 1.8 after being treated with fresh frozen plasma and vitamin K. After one week of stable INR levels he was discharged. Approximately 2 weeks after discharge he was readmitted to the hospital with an INR of 11.55. After this hospital admission, his pharmacist counselled him again on the possible interaction of cannabis and warfarin. The patient decided to stop using medical cannabis for his depression. In the following months his INR stayed between 1.08 and 4.40.[290]

Pharmacodynamic and cannabis interaction case reports of this severity are not common, so aggregate case report conclusions are difficult to reach with certainty. Rather than being evidence for absolute contraindication, case reports such as these should foster additional research and be used as indicators for more detailed benefit-risk analysis by the patient, physician, and pharmacist team. Pharmacists should treat cannabis like any other prescription medicine when they are counseling patients. By including cannabis in the normal interaction checks, these types of serious events can be minimized. In states where patients are using medical cannabis, the pharmacist should include cannabis interactions in their normal counseling points to ensure the patient is aware of the risk.

Chapter 17: Addiction and Abuse

There is no shame in using cannabis medicine to aid in health and healing. Just like other prescribed medicine, for some conditions cannabis may assist the healing process and no longer be needed, while other conditions may require regular and ongoing use.

It is possible to become mentally addicted to cannabis. While cannabis is significantly less addictive compared to cigarettes, alcohol, prescription opiate painkillers, or drugs like cocaine and heroin, the risk of addiction to cannabis should be taken seriously. Steps should be taken to avoid unnecessary dependency issues.

Addiction evolves when a person cannot resist the desire for something despite the continued use of it causing a known problem or problems to the person. Addiction causes problems with:

- Relationships
- Ability to support oneself and/or family
- Self-image
- Health

If relationships, job performance, self-image, and/or health are suffering rather than improving, the cannabis medicine is being misused or used too much. Continued, compulsive use of cannabis medicine in such a manner points to an addiction problem. If cannabis medicine use is causing these problems and a patient is struggling to have self-control regarding its use, the patient-pharmacist-physician team (along with the patient's community support system) should work to end the use of cannabis and develop a different plan for health and healing.

Chapter 18: Tolerance

By nature, cannabis can build up tolerance in the body. A compulsive need to feel greater and greater physical or psychotropic effects through increased consumption (that is not lending itself to improved health, self-image, ability to perform tasks to provide for oneself and/or family, or relationships) is addiction. A need to consume more and more cannabis to achieve relief that is helping a patient maintain health or heal (that is not negatively impacting their life) is an issue of cannabis tolerance in the body. To avoid cannabis tolerance build-up, a patient should:

- Follow the low and slow medicating protocol
- Avoid over-medicating
- In instances when cannabis medicine is needed for a chronic condition, work with their pharmacist and physician to create a plan for quarterly cannabis detoxes (this plan should include alternatives to cannabis for symptom relief during the detox)
  - Weaning off period over 5-9 days
  - Cannabis abstinence period of 9-14 days
  - Reintroduce cannabis using the low and slow medicating protocol

Chapter 19: CBD and Industrial Hemp Cannabis

CBD vs. THC

It has become a common belief that the cannabinoid THC is psychoactive/psychotropic/high-inducing and CBD is non-psychoactive/non-psychotropic/does not produce a high. While CBD does not generate the levels of euphoria (and sometimes dysphoria) that THC does, research shows that CBD has antipsychotic, anti anxiety, and antidepressant capabilities. Contrary to common public discourse, CBD is a mood-altering chemical. It just does not alter a person in the same way, and/or to the degree, THC does.

The false dichotomy between CBD and THC has created a legislative culture where CBD-only laws are seen as safer, and legalization efforts for full spectrum medicine have been met with greater concern. Similarly, great efforts have been made to separate medical and recreational cannabis from industrial hemp. Medical and recreational cannabis and industrial hemp are all cannabis. In each case, the plant has been selected or bred for different phytochemical and physical qualities.

Nomenclature

There is a significant amount of misinformation, both purposeful and unintended, about CBD oil. The confusion starts with nomenclature. Consumers are forced to try to differentiate between "hemp seed oil," "hemp CBD oil," and "High CBD oil" to name a few of the most common. All of these oils are derived from the cannabis plant; however, they are processed from different parts of the plant, have different phytochemical makeups (thus, different health benefits), and have varying degrees of legality.

It is important to understand the difference between legal definitions of cannabis and industrial hemp. Industrial hemp has less than 0.3% of the cannabinoid THC and has historically been cultivated to produce more seeds and stalk than resin. Medical and adult-use cannabis has varying degrees of cannabinoid content (though, usually higher in THC) and has historically been cultivated to produce larger resinous flowers known as buds. There is now a trend in industrial hemp production to grow hemp plants more similarly to the way adult-use cannabis is grown. This allows a much greater CBD yield.

Industrial Hemp Seed Oil

Hemp seed oil is made from pressing seeds of industrial hemp. Isolated hemp seed oil contains nearly no cannabinoids, so it is not used to produce CBD oil (though it is sometimes combined with industrial hemp CBD oil to assist the consistency and supplement the nutritional content). Hemp seed oil does have a variety of health benefits either as a consumed supplement or as a topical. It is 3:1 ratio of Omega-6 to Omega-3 mercury free fatty acids.[291] It contains sterols, alcohols, tocopherols, Gamma-linolenic acid (GLA), vitamin E, and 25% of the oil is comprised of a complete protein source offering all of the essential amino acids.[292] Because of this makeup, it is used as a supplement for heart health, inflammation, hormone balancing, and immune health.[293] It is also used topically for acne, eczema, and as a moisturizer. Hemp seed oil containing the most nutritional value is cold-pressed and unrefined. Refined hemp seed oil is most commonly used for body care products, but the more refined the oil, the lesser degree of phytochemical bioavailability there is for presumed health benefits.

Industrial Hemp CBD Oil

Industrial hemp CBD-rich oil comes from the resinous trichomes of industrial hemp plants. The oil can be full extract (contains all of the extracted plant material with only the solvent removed), full spectrum (contains an array of cannabinoids, terpenes and lesser phytochemicals, but the solvent and some plant materials like chlorophyll and most lipids have been removed), or the oil can be distilled down to a CBD isolate form (only contains CBD and no other phytochemicals—usually takes the form of a crystal or powder).

CBD-rich industrial hemp products either come from industrial hemp sourced outside of the United States (most commonly Eastern Europe and China), or from industrial hemp sourced within the United States under the 2014 Farm Bill Industrial Hemp Pilot Research Programs. As previously discussed, only CBD-rich industrial hemp products from United States pilot programs are legal. Companies that source CBD outside of the United States claim their CBD is sourced from seed and stalk in order to try to skirt the CSA, but it is unlikely that they are not using the resinous flower of the cannabis plant to source the CBD. The DEA has communicated to these companies that they are not operating under the legal CBD framework, however little has been done to shut the companies down.

If a company is sourcing overseas compliant oils, the process to extract enough CBD oil from the stalk and seed requires large amounts of hemp. Also, it usually involves solvents such as hexane and thinning compounds like propylene glycol (that may convert to formaldehyde when heated/inhaled).[294] In the rare cases of finding solventless/additive free European or Chinese industrial hemp CBD oil, there is also a significant chance for accumulated toxins in the oil due to cannabis being a bioremediator—it absorbs toxins from the soil. As the plant is processed for oil, the toxins in the plant are concentrated and passed to the consumer. In addition, these CBD oils often lack other phytochemicals in the plant that create a more therapeutic entourage effect.[295]

Legality aside, some of the CBD-rich products with European and Chinese sourced crude-oil CBD or isolate, are problematic due to production and processing practices that can be taxing on the environment, issues of contaminants such as pesticides and heavy metals, and lack of transparency regarding all aspects of production.

CBD-rich Medical Cannabis

That brings us to high-CBD medical cannabis. This concentrate and flower is derived from what is commonly termed marijuana, but marijuana plants that have been bred to possess more of the cannabinoid CBD. CBD-rich medical cannabis will have various ratios of CBD to THC depending on the strain or compounding of the product. Legally, it can only be grown, processed, and distributed within individual states that have legalized the cultivation, processing, distribution, and possession of medical and/or recreational cannabis. Research is indicating that cannabis with CBD and THC tends to be more efficacious in treating a majority of disease states. While the more benign nature of CBD has created an accepted culture of CBD-only philosophies, access to THC is important. We are learning that CBD may offset the psychotropic effects of THC, which help patients access the other plethora of symptom relieving properties THC has while decreasing what many feel is a negative side effect from THC of feeling "high."

Considerations for Consuming Industrial Hemp CBD Products

Choosing the Right Product

The variety of industrial hemp cbd-rich products on the market make choosing the correct product overwhelming. The same initial and ongoing self-assessment is needed for CBD medicating as for broader medical cannabis medicating. Identify the symptoms you have that you are looking to relieve, consider the type of products available, and consider the modes of consumption for the products. Products will vary in the symptoms they can best target based on the phytochemical makeup of the product and how it can be delivered. CBD flower, vape-pen, alcohol tincture, or glycerine tincture will provide more rapid relief but will have shorter duration. An ingested full extract, full spectrum, or isolate oil will take a little longer to relieve symptoms but will have a longer duration. A topical will target location-specific symptoms at the dermis level but will not aid in overall ECS supplementation. Not all products share the same cannabinoids, terpenes and lesser phytochemicals, so if one product does not work that isn't always an indication that no product will work.

Consider the below set of criteria when looking at different brands:

- Produced under a United States Industrial Hemp Pilot Research Program
- Organic/Sustainable production principles are used in cultivation, processing and packaging
- Third-party testing is transparent and accessible
- Free from pesticides, mold, mildew, and metals
- Full spectrum—containing as many of the phytochemicals in the plant as possible
  - CO2 Extraction techniques are very common, but BHO and alcohol solvent techniques tend to provide a more full spectrum
    - If derived from a solvent extraction method, tested to prove no residual solvents present

Dosing

The same low and slow dosing protocol should be followed as was described for broader medical cannabis. Begin with five-to-ten milligrams of CBD once a day for three to five days and, by adding a dose every three to five days, work up to five-to-ten milligrams of CBD every four-to-six hours. At that point determine if all three daily doses are needed or if you can scale back. Conversely, you may want to add more milligrams per dose if you are not seeing the relief desired. Acute symptoms, may be better treated with a larger dose of CBD in the range of 50-200 milligrams. Generally, it is recommended to try to take the smallest dose possible as few times as possible to slow tolerance buildup, but each person is different in dosage needs. Utilizing self-assessment tools will help dial in the dose. As described earlier in this book, quarterly detoxes are suggested to keep tolerance build up to a minimum.

Side Effects

Potential side effects of CBD include becoming light-headed (or dizzy), warming of the cheeks, dry mouth, lowering of blood pressure, lowering of blood sugar, and drowsiness (or sedation). Side effects are amplified with large doses, especially the sedative effect. While CBD is generally benign and safe to use, persons with complex medical conditions and those taking other prescriptions (especially blood sugar, blood pressure, blood thinner medications, and medications for severe mental health disorders) should consult with their health care team to make the proper risk assessment decisions.

Other Uses of Industrial Hemp Cannabis

Hemp was a viable crop in the United States prior to the 1930s, mostly for fiber but also fuel. It had a resurgence during World War II when US hemp imports were interrupted and was still seen as distinct from marijuana until the CSA of 1970. Like medical and recreational cannabis, industrial hemp has suffered multiple suppressions due to successful lobbying efforts by competing industries and political agendas.[296]

If our own history of the efficacy of hemp wasn't enough to support full legalization of industrial hemp, we have international examples of agriculturally and commercially successful industrial hemp programs. These programs are predominately successful due to supplying raw, refined, and processed materials to the United States for consumption. It is estimated that the US makes up 60% of the sales market for industrial hemp, consuming around $600Million in industrial hemp derived products. If global projections follow US projections, the total global market is projected to reach $3 Billion by 2020.[297]

China is the world's single largest hemp producing and exporting country, mostly of hemp textiles and related products, as well as a major supplier of these products to the United States:

China reportedly produced nearly 80 million pounds on about 30,000 acres, accounting for about one-fifth of global production. [...] Canada is also a major supplier of U.S. hemp imports, particularly of hemp-based foods and food ingredients and other related imported products. [...] Total production across all European countries is reported at nearly 250 million pounds on more than 70,000 acres, accounting for about two-thirds of the U.N.-reported global production. Most of this production is in Western Europe. The European Union (EU) has an active hemp market, with production in most member nations. Production is centered in France, the Netherlands, Lithuania, and Romania. Many EU countries lifted their bans on hemp production in the 1990s and, until recently, also subsidized the production of "flax and hemp" under the EU's Common Agricultural Policy. Most EU production is of hurds, seeds, and fibers. Other non-EU European countries with reported hemp production include Russia, Ukraine, and Switzerland. Other countries with active hemp grower and consumer markets are Australia, New Zealand, India, Japan, Korea, Turkey, Egypt, Chile, and Thailand.[298]

There are over 30,000 products that use hemp including:

- Food: hemp seeds, milk, and ice cream
- Supplements: hemp seed oil, CBD oil, and protein powder
- Body care products: soaps, lotions, and moisturizers
- Fiber: textiles, biofuel, building material, paper, cordage, and plastics

There are several advantages of growing and processing hemp compared to other resources:

- Hemp is naturally resistant to most pests and grows densely resulting in reduced use of herbicides or pesticides
- Hemp remediates and revitalizes the soil – it pulls toxins from the soil while also aerating the soil, redepositing carbon

dioxide
- Hemp grows in a variety of climates and soil types
- Hemp requires less water than most crops to grow
- Hemp fights global warming through the reduction of atmospheric CO2 at a rate four times faster than trees
- Hemp is superior to cotton, wood, and concrete in strength, renewability, and environmental footprint
- Hemp biodiesel is the cleanest ethanol to produce and burn[299]

Hemp programs in the states are gaining momentum. Colorado and Kentucky are great examples.[300] [301] As shown above, hemp is comparatively an easy crop to grow. We also know the plethora of applications for the plant. Yet, in order for the industry to take off, there is a significant need for new technologies, more processors, and new manufacturing capabilities. This provides further evidence that hemp can be a significant boon to the economy. Many articles quoting stateside hemp farmers and many hemp farmers we have talked with indicate that they need access to new hemp-specific farm equipment, more processing companies as an outlet for their crop, and more companies willing to invest in manufacturing technologies that would produce more hemp products.[302]

Chapter 20: Conclusion

Throughout history, cannabis has been cultivated for agricultural, medical, industrial, social and spiritual purposes. Historical hindsight affords humanity the perspective to see how various choices we have made, including consumptive choices, have impacted us. Research has further deepened our understanding of whether certain foods and drugs are beneficial, harmful, or potentially have benefits that may outweigh risks for certain people.

Considering the historical perspective of cannabis and the current scientific understanding, there is evidence of thousands of years of cannabis consumption without great harm. Despite roadblocks to research during the last 100 years of cannabis prohibition, the surmounting research we do have indicates that cannabis is non-toxic, non-lethal, and has medical benefit. While cannabis may have numbered negative side effects, the negative side effects of cannabis are not greater than some over-the-counter medications, many prescription drugs, and definitely alcohol.

It wasn't until recent history (early 1900s) that the use of cannabis became outlawed and subject to controversy. Cannabis became a pawn in a socio-political power play with additional capitalist undertones that marred it as a highly addictive and dangerous drug. Ironically, cannabis prohibition sentiment oscillates between two competing sentiments—both arguing cannabis is equally dangerous to society for two very different reasons. One sentiment is that cannabis is and aggressively lethal illicit drug that brings with it violence and mayhem. Simultaneously, cannabis is argued as dangerous because it creates lazy, thoughtless "stoners" leaching from society and not contributing to the workforce. Neither are true.

Despite political and social movements of the last 50 years, in which subjects of oppression have made visible the tactics of those in power to maintain control and stay in power—cannabis advocates have not been able to shed enough light on the usurpation of the cannabis narrative as a power-play rather than actuated in truth and science. Cannabis use remains a feared and controversial topic to this day in spite of historical context and scientific findings. With more than half of states allowing some form of cannabis legalization, there are still many against the use of cannabis for any reason.

The main arguments in support of continued cannabis prohibition are that cannabis is a dangerous drug in-and-of-itself, there is not ample evidence of the medical value of cannabis, more research is needed, legalization will endanger our youth, cannabis causes psychosis, cannabis is a gateway drug to even more dangerous drugs, legalization will lead to rampant drugged driving, and an intoxicated workforce will negatively impact productivity. This primer has presented evidence that, while cannabis has side effects to be considered, it is non-toxic, non-lethal, and safer than some over-the-counter medications, many prescription drugs, and most certainly alcohol. The evidence of the medical value of cannabis has been presented. While we conclude that more research is warranted, there is enough research to support rescheduling cannabis in order to increase access to research potential. Additionally, once the veil of Drug War propaganda is removed, there is a strong argument for descheduling rather than rescheduling. Little time was spent in this book discussing the remaining prohibition arguments. Evidence used in support of these arguments has common themes: biased research, cherry-picking data, and findings based on correlation instead of causation. A more thorough investigation of the dominant prohibition talking points lead to these actual findings:

- **Cannabis and youth:** recent states with medical marijuana laws had 1.1 percent fewer teenage cannabis smokers than states without such laws:

  Interestingly, the longer medical marijuana laws had been on the books, the less likely teenagers were to use pot -- about 9 percent lower odds in states with laws five years old or fewer, compared with 32 percent lower odds if the law had been in effect for more than 10 years.[303]

- **Cannabis and psychosis:** research does not conclude that cannabis causes a psychosis disorder—rather both early use and heavy use of cannabis are more likely in individuals with a vulnerability to psychosis.[304]

- **Cannabis and brain function:** preliminary evidence out of Harvard Medical School suggests that medical marijuana may not impair, and in many cases, may actually improve executive functioning in adults.[305]
- **Cannabis and the gateway theory:**

> Research simply does not support the theory that marijuana is a "gateway" drug – that is, one whose use results in an increased likelihood of using "more serious" drugs such as cocaine and heroin. However, this flawed gateway effect is one of the principal reasons cited in defense of laws prohibiting the use or possession of marijuana. Research shows that marijuana could more accurately be described as a "terminus" drug because the vast majority of people who use marijuana do not go on to use other illicit drugs.[1,2] Marijuana has never been proven to have an actual "gateway effect."[3] However, a more critical interpretation of this and further research suggests that those who use drugs may instead have an underlying propensity to do so that is not specific to any one drug.[4,5,6][306]

- **Cannabis and drugged driving:** a new study conducted at the University of Iowa's National Advanced Driving Simulator (NADS) has found drivers testing at the common legal limit of THC at, or below, 5 ng/mL caused almost no impairment. Not until blood concentrations of 13.1 ug/L THC did drivers show impairment. That impairment was increased weaving similar to drivers at most state's legal limit of .08 breath alcohol concentration. The drivers were assessed on weaving within the lane, how often the car left the lane, and the speed of the weaving. Drivers with only alcohol in their systems showed impairment in all three areas while those strictly under the influence of vaporized cannabis only demonstrated problems weaving within the lane.[307] Additionally:

141

A final study, published in the American Journal of Public Health, explored the same relationships as the NBER paper but using a longer time period (1985–2014), during which more states had enacted medical marijuana laws. This study also added the condition that dispensaries were operational. Again, the authors found that states with MML laws had lower traffic fatality rates. On average, traffic fatalities decreased by 10.8% following the enactment of MML. However, the effect varied considerably from state to state: seven states experienced fatality decreases while in two states (Rhode Island and Connecticut) MML laws were associated with an increase in fatalities. Meanwhile, contrary to the findings of the previous NBER study, the presence of operational dispensaries was associated with a decrease in accident fatalities.[308]

Cannabis prohibitionists regularly use recent Colorado vehicle accident findings as evidence for grave consequences of cannabis drugged driving, but a closer look at the statistics shows only a three percent increase in collisions and no increase in fatal collisions in Colorado since recreational cannabis has been legalized:

Pre–recreational marijuana legalization annual changes in motor vehicle crash fatality rates for Washington and Colorado were similar to those for the control states. Post–recreational marijuana legalization changes in motor vehicle crash fatality rates for Washington and Colorado also did not significantly differ from those for the control states (adjusted difference-in-differences coefficient=+0.2 fatalities/billion vehicle miles traveled; 95% confidence interval=−0.4, +0.9).[309]

Additionally, statistics describing a steep leap in increased cannabis in the system of drivers involved in fatal car accidents does not provide additional evidence that cannabis intoxication was the cause of the collision. It is common sense to think that a state where cannabis is legal for adult-use would find cannabis more commonly in the system of victims, but (as cannabis remains measurable in the body after intoxication ends) to the causal link of cannabis consumption with traffic fatalities falls short.

- **Cannabis and productivity:** a recent study suggests that cannabis legalization does not negatively impact worker attendance. With what is known about cannabis legalization and reduction in alcohol, pharmaceutical, and non-prescribed opioid consumption, it is likely we will see a healthier and more present workforce versus the contrary.[310]

The remaining three counter-arguments against cannabis legalization (that cannabis is a dangerous drug in-and-of-itself, there is not ample evidence of the medical value of cannabis, and research is needed) were the focus of this book. Drugs approved by the FDA have gone through rigorous studies showing patient safety in long term use and repeatable, consistent effects from well-controlled, unbiased, blinded, and randomized drug trials. Critics citing the lack of wide acceptance from qualified experts and concrete scientific evidence to support denial of the legitimacy of cannabis-as-medicine are making claims that are not spurious. Cannabis-as-medicine does not have the same scientific backing and repeatable results as FDA approved medications. There are no major medical professional organizations that approve and support the use of medical cannabis. The FDA has not approved any dispensary cannabis product due to variations in potency and lack of consistent standards. All of these are valid arguments against the use of cannabis-as-medicine. However, these claims combined with current Federal law does not remedy the ability to legitimate medical cannabis in the way the trending research indicates we ought to.

Evidence to support the re-, or de-, scheduling of cannabis from the CSA requires the approval of the federal government to conduct research. Before embarking on a new clinical study, researchers must get the approval from a litany of organizations which may include the National Institute on Drug Abuse (NIDA), the FDA, the DEA, institutional review boards, state level departments, state boards of

143

medical examiners, and potential funders. If any of these groups rejects the research, the project can be delayed and/or shelved. The NIDA is the government group that has been tasked with determining the cause and effects of drug addiction and abuse; their focus is not on finding therapeutic uses for drugs, but rather determining the consequences of drug use and abuse on individual and public health. As such, less than 20% of the cannabis research funded by NIDA in 2015 focused on the therapeutic benefits of cannabis.

Supply issues plague researchers as well. Federally, the only place allowed to cultivate cannabis as defined under the CSA is the University of Mississippi. Researchers must gain approval from the NIDA and then request cannabis from the University of Mississippi. Historically, the quality of the product produced at the University of Mississippi has not been equivalent to the products being cultivated and sold at dispensaries. Due to changes in supply and demand stemming from production restrictions and research approval, product is often stored frozen for long periods before being sent to researchers. This can affect the potency of the product. Due to only being cultivated by one entity, the variety of products do not match what is available to the public in medical and/or recreational markets. As a result of increased pressure from researchers, steps have been taken to remedy some of these issues, but changes have been slow. The NIDA has instructed the University of Mississippi to look at cultivating various THC concentration plants, and the DEA has agreed to increase the number of licenses allowed for federally legal cannabis cultivators for research purposes (although at this time, no other licenses have been awarded).

After a study receives the approval of the appropriate agencies, groups, or offices, and is able to obtain adequate product from the NIDA, there is still the hurdle of "blinding" patients. For a study to be generally accepted by the medical community, the participants must be "blinded". This means a study participant should not be aware if they are getting active drug, in this case cannabis, or a placebo. The NIDA does provide a very low dose cannabis product (0.001% THC) that still has terpenes intact to retain the smell of cannabis. Despite this, it is often difficult to truly have patients blind to their

144

arm of treatment due to the psychoactive component of cannabis. This puts researchers between a rock and a hard place. If researchers do not assess whether patients were properly blinded, or if it is later determined that the patients were not properly blinded, the research findings will not be accepted by the medical community. Without wide acceptance of the medical community, national medical organizations are not going to come forward and support the use of cannabis for medical purposes.

These hurdles make it nearly impossible for adequate research to be performed on cannabis-as-medicine. The status of cannabis as a schedule I entity ensures that these hurdles will remain in place until the DEA reschedules cannabis. The National Academies of Science, Medicine, and Engineering states that "In short, such barriers represent a public health problem."[311] Despite cannabis being stuck in this revolving door scenario, the limited research performed in the United States, extensive research going on outside of the United States, and 25 years of patients medicating with cannabis under various state sanctioned programs affords us a foundation of information about cannabis-as-medicine to assess risk/benefit analysis and apply sensible protocols for incorporating medical cannabis into symptom relief therapies.

* For the most recent discussions of the political landscapes of cannabis, please visit the blog section at www.phytopharmd.com

* For the most recent discussions on cannabis production, please visit the blog section at www.WholePlantTechnologies.com

About the Authors

Joshua T. Winningham, Pharm.D

Josh Winningham has been a practicing pharmacist in the state of Arkansas since graduating from the University of Arkansas for Medical Sciences College of Pharmacy in 2011. Throughout his career, Josh has gained experience in community, hospital, healthcare system, and nuclear pharmacy. His current responsibilities include overseeing the clinical services and medication therapy management programs for his pharmacy and acting as the preceptor for the intern program. He is based out of Cabot, AR where he lives with his wife and their two children.

Josh has partnered with Whole Plant Technologies to launch PhytoPharm.D—a medical cannabis pharmacist consulting company. PhytoPharm.D offers the medical cannabis industry 50 combined years of pharmacy and cannabis cultivation, processing, and dispensing experience. Merging pharmaceutical standards of compounding and dispensing with medical cannabis knowledge and dispensary experience, PhytoPharm.D offers a patient first, science driven, holistic approach to education and supporting medical cannabis patients.

Abigail M. Testaberg

Abbie Testaberg is the co-founder and COO of Whole Plant Technologies—a mediumless aeroponic cultivation system manufacturer, production facility design, and business startup consulting firm. Ms. Testaberg co-founded and collaboratively executed the startup of PhytoPharm.D—a consumer and dispensary education company with a pharmacist driven approach. In addition, Abbie is a co-founder and owner/operator of Kinni Hemp Company—cultivating, processing, and producing CBD rich hemp products under the Wisconsin Industrial Hemp Pilot Research Program. Ms. Testaberg focuses her efforts on driving science, innovation, and education in the cannabis realm, while maintaining a mindfulness toward the holistic integrity of patients and environmentally sustainable business choices.

Jesse Long

Jesse Long grew up in the Cannabis hotbed that is Oregon, and was generally able to develop his relationship with the plant without stigma or reprisal. After attending the University of Oregon, he became a budtender during the medical-only epoch of Oregon legal cannabis and witnessed first-hand the transition of cannabis in Oregon to full adult-use legalization. Jesse has subsequent experience as a cultivation distribution manager and operations management experience for Whole Plant Technologies and now Green Source Gardens - a leading permaculture cannabis cultivation farm in Oregon. With a passion for learning and disseminating that knowledge, Jesse seeks to normalize the use of cannabis in our society. Due in part to his Political Science background, he has a fascination with the political and legal dynamics that are allowing the full potential of Cannabis to be scientifically substantiated and the transformative potential of its by-products realized.

Buck Duncan

Buck Duncan received his education in horticulture from the University of Wisconsin - River Falls. He has ten years of horticulture grow management experience, which includes nursery and greenhouse operations, plant management and logistics management. Buck worked with Whole Plant Technologies as the Head of Cultivation and now owns and operates his own hemp farm under the Wisconsin Industrial Hemp Pilot Research Program.

Jody Testaberg

Jody Testaberg's passion for cannabis cultivation and grow technologies pushed him to seek out education in historic practices and innovative techniques throughout strategic growing cultures both nationally and internationally. Twenty years of progressive growing experience, management roles in construction and manufacturing, and owner/operator entrepreneurship afforded Jody the expertise that launched Whole Plant Technologies. Whole Plant Technologies manufactures, installs, and trains the use of a mediumless aeroponic cultivation system made from FDA approved food grade plastic that is reusable and 30% more profitable compared to other industry standard grow systems such as soil, coco coir drip irrigation, and rock wool. Whole Plant Technologies offers vertically integrated consulting services including business planning, facility design, cultivation and processing SOP's and training, and application and licensure support. Whole Plant Technologies values a patient-first approach emphasizing safe, accessible and affordable cannabis without compromising quality. Ownership in PhytoPharm.D and Kinni Hemp Company allows Whole Plant Technologies to support their values of safe, accessible, affordable and quality cannabis.

Additional Resources

Please visit the following websites for more information:

www.phytopharmd.com

www.wholeplanttechnologies.com

www.wholeplanthemp.com

www.kinnihempco.com

Endnotes

1   Bentley JH, Ziegler HF, Streets-Salter H. Traditions and Encounters: A Global Perspective on the Past. Boston, MA: McGraw-Hill Education; 2015:15-19.

2   Clarke RC, Merlin MD, Cannabis: Evolution and Ethnobotany. Berkeley, CA: University of California Press; 2013:24.

3   Merline MD. COVER ARTICLE. Archeological evidence for the tradition of psychoactive plant use in the old world. Economic Botany. 2003;57(3):296.

4   Merline MD. COVER ARTICLE. Archeological evidence for the tradition of psychoactive plant use in the old world. Economic Botany. 2003;57(3):312-13

5   Abel EL. Marijuana - The First Twelve Thousand Years. New York, NY: Plenum Press; 1980:5-7.

6   Merline MD. Cover Article. Archeological evidence for the tradition of psychoactive plant use in the old world. Economic Botany. 2003;57(3):316.

7   Courtwright DT. Forces of Habit: Drugs and the Making of the Modern World. USA: First Harvard University Press; 2002:41.

8   Deitch R. Hemp: American History Revisited: The Plant with a Divided History. New York, NY: Algora Pub; 2003:25-27

9   Library of Congress. Digital Collection. George Washington Papers. Washington and the New Agriculture. https://www.loc.gov/collections/george-washington-papers/articles-and-essays/introduction-to-the-diaries-of-george-washington/washington-and-the-new-agriculture/. Accessed February 25, 2018.

10   "Washington and the New Agriculture | Introduction to the Diaries of George Washington | Articles and Essays | George Washington Papers | Digital Collections | Library of Congress." The Library of Congress. https://www.loc.gov/collections/george-washington-papers/articles-and-essays/introduction-to-the-diaries-of-george-washington/washington-and-the-new-agriculture/. Accessed October 15, 2018.

11   Suman C, Lata H, ElSohly MA. Cannabis Sativa L.: Botany and Biotechnology. Oxford, MS: Springer International Publishing, 2017:26.

12   Duvall CS. Decriminalization doesn't address marijuana's standing as a drug of the poor. The Conversation. https://theconversation.com/decriminalization-doesnt-address-marijuanas-standing-as-a-drug-of-the-poor-42345.   Published September 19, 2018. Accessed October 19, 2018.

13   Lee MA. Smoke Signals: a Social History of Marijuana: Medical, Recreational, and Scientific. New York, NY: Scribner; 2013:39.

14   McKenna GJ. The Current Status of Medical Marijuana in the United States. Hawaii J Med Public Health. 2014;73(4):105-108.

15   Musto DF. Opium, Cocaine and Marijuana in American History. Scientific American. 1991;265(1):40-47. doi:10.1038/scientificamerican0791-40.

16   McKenna GJ. The Current Status of Medical Marijuana in the United States. Hawaii J Med Public Health. 2014;73(4):105-108.

17   Schneider A, Ingram H. Social Construction of Target Populations: Implications for Politics and Policy. American Political Science Review. 1993;87(02):334-347. doi:10.2307/2939044.

18   Thornton M. The Economics of Prohibition. Salt Lake City: University of Utah Press; 1991:11.

19   Zheng Y. The Social Life of Opium in China. Cambridge: Cambridge University Press; 2005:97.

20   Reksulak M, Hillman AL, Razzolini L, Shughart WF. The Elgar Companion to Public Choice. Northampton, MA: Edward Elgar; 2013:307-330.

21   Thornton M. The Economics of Prohibition. Salt Lake City: University of Utah Press; 1991:59-60.

22   Pederson WD, Wolf TP, Daynes BW. Franklin D. Roosevelt and Congress: the New Deal and Its Aftermath. Armonk, New York: Sharpe; 2001:29-34.

23   Thornton M. The Economics of Prohibition. Salt Lake City: University of Utah Press; 1991:66-67.

24   Gray M. Drug Crazy: How We Got into This Mess and How We Can Get Out. New York, NY: Routledge; 2000:75-76.

25   Kyvig DE. Repealing National Prohibition. Kent, OH: Kent State University Press; 2000:6.

26   Stewart J. "The Economics of American Farm Unrest, 1865-1900." EH.Net Encyclopedia, edited by Robert Whaples. February 10, 2008. URL http://eh.net/encyclopedia/the-economics-of-american-farm-unrest-1865-1900/

27   Kyvig DE. Repealing National Prohibition. Kent, OH: Kent State University Press; 2000:8.

28   Kyvig DE. Repealing National Prohibition. Kent, OH: Kent State University Press; 2000:11.

29   Blocker JS. Did Prohibition Really Work? Alcohol Prohibition as a Public Health Innovation. American Journal of Public Health. 2006;96(2):233-243. doi:10.2105/ajph.2005.065409.

30   Bewley-Taylor DR. The United States and International Drug Control: 1909-1997. London: Pinter; 1999:6.

31   Jensen EL, Gerber J, Mosher C. Social Consequences of the War on Drugs: the Legacy of Failed Policy. Criminal Justice Policy Review. 2004;15(1):100-121.

32   UNODC, World Drug Report 2010 (United Nations Publication, Sales No. E.10.XI.13).

33   War on Drugs: Report of the Global Commission on Drug Policy 2011. Geneva, Switzerland: Global Commission on Drug Policy. https://www.globalcommissionondrugs.org/wp-content/themes/gcdp_v1/pdf/Global_

Commission_Report_English.pdf. Accessed February 26, 2018.

34   National Institute on Drug Abuse. National Trends Based on the National Survey on Drug Use and Health 2013. https://www.drugabuse.gov/publications/drugfacts/nationwide-trends. Revised June 2015. Accessed February 26, 2018.

35   Payan T. A War That Can't Be Won: Binational Perspectives on the War on Drugs. Tucson: Univ. of Arizona Press; 2013:33-58.

36   War on Drugs: Report of the Global Commission on Drug Policy 2011. Geneva, Switzerland: Global Commission on Drug Policy. https://www.globalcommissionondrugs.org/wp-content/themes/gcdp_v1/pdf/Global_Commission_Report_English.pdf. Accessed February 26, 2018.

37   Room R. Cannabis Policy: Moving beyond Stalemate. Oxford: Oxford University Press; 2010:85.

38   Boire RG, Feeney K. Medical Marijuana Law. Berkeley, CA: Ronin; 2007:23-25.

39   Boire RG, Feeney K. Medical Marijuana Law. Berkeley, CA: Ronin; 2007:25-26.

40   Boire RG, Feeney K. Medical Marijuana Law. Berkeley, CA: Ronin; 2007:26-28.

41   31 Legal Medical Marijuana States and DC - Medical Marijuana - ProCon.org. Should marijuana be a medical option? https://medicalmarijuana.procon.org/view.resource.php?resourceID=000881. Accessed October 19, 2018.

42   Wallach PA, Rauch J. Bootleggers, Baptists, bureaucrats, and bongs: How special interests will shape marijuana legalization. Brookings. https://www.brookings.edu/research/bootleggers-baptists-bureaucrats-and-bongs-how-special-interests-will-shape-marijuana-legalization/. Published July 28, 2016. Accessed October 19, 2018.

43   Borchardt D. Beer Industry Could Lose $2 Billion From Legal Marijuana. Forbes. https://www.forbes.com/sites/debraborchardt/2017/03/13/beer-industry-could-lose-2-billion-from-legal-marijuana/#30c15e5428c1. Published March 13, 2017. Accessed October 19, 2018.

44   Baggio M, Chong A, Kwon S. Marijuana and Alcohol Evidence Using Border Analysis and Retail Sales Data (August 23, 2018). Available at SSRN: https://ssrn.com/abstract=3063288 or http://dx.doi.org/10.2139/ssrn.3063288

45   Close K. Legal Marijuana Hurts Beer Sales | Money. Time. http://time.com/money/4592317/legal-marijuana-beer-sales/. Published December 6, 2016. Accessed October 19, 2018.

46   Wallach P, Rauch J. Bootleggers, Baptists, Bureaucrats, and Bongs: How special interests will shape marijuana legalization. Center for Effective Public Management at Brookings. June 2016:1-22. https://www.brookings.edu/wp-content/uploads/2016/07/bootleggers.pdf. Accessed February 26, 2018.

47   Bradford AC, Bradford WD. Medical Marijuana Laws Reduce Prescription Medication Use In Medicare Part D. Health Affairs. 2016;35(7):1230-1236. https://www.healthaffairs.org/doi/10.1377/hlthaff.2015.1661.

48   Fang L. Leading Anti-Marijuana Academics Are Paid by Painkiller Drug Companies. Vice. https://www.vice.com/en_us/article/4w7byq/leading-anti-marijuana-academics-are-paid-by-painkiller-drug-companies. Published August 27, 2014. Accessed October 22, 2018.

49   Pauly M, Gilson D, Steffen A, Lanard N. A brief history of America's corporate-run prison industry. Mother Jones. https://www.motherjones.com/politics/2016/06/history-of-americas-private-prison-industry-timeline/. Published June 23, 2017. Accessed October 22, 2018.

50   King RS, Mauer M. The war on marijuana: The transformation of the war on drugs in the 1990s. Harm Reduction Journal. February 2006. https://harmreductionjournal.biomedcentral.com/articles/10.1186/1477-7517-3-6. Accessed October 22, 2018.

51   Feinstein, other Democrats accept donations from architect of Arizona immigration law. https://dailycaller.com/2010/11/01/feinstein-other-democrats-accept-donations-from-architect-of-arizona-immigration-law/. Accessed October 22, 2018..

52   The Top Five Special Interest Groups Lobbying To Keep Marijuana Illegal. Republic Report. https://www.republicreport.org/2012/marijuana-lobby-illegal. Published May 16, 2012. Accessed July 4, 2018.

53   Wallach P, Rauch J. Bootleggers, Baptists, Bureaucrats, and Bongs: How special interests will shape marijuana legalization. Center for Effective Public Management at Brookings. June 2016:1-22. https://www.brookings.edu/wp-content/uploads/2016/07/bootleggers.pdf. Accessed February 26, 2018.

54   Doughton RL, Woodward WC. The Marihuana Tax Act of 1937. Schaffer Library of Drug Policy. http://www.druglibrary.org/Schaffer/hemp/taxact/woodward.htm. Published May 4, 1937. Accessed July 4, 2018.

55   The La Guardia Committee Report. La Guardia Committee Report, The Marihuana Problem in the City of New York, Mayor's Committee on Marihuana, by the New York Academy of Medicine. Schaffer Library of Drug Policy. http://druglibrary.net/schaffer/Library/studies/lag/lagmenu.htm. Accessed October 22, 2018.

56   Booth M. Cannabis: a History. London: Transworld Digital; 2011 https://books.google.com/s?id=ccITBwAAQBAJ&lpg=PA205&dq=laguardiareportcannabis&pg=PA205#v=onepage&q=laguardiareportcannabis&f=false. Accessed July 4, 2018.

57   Boire RG, Feeney K. Medical Marijuana Law. Berkeley, CA: Ronin; 2007: 21.

58   The Report of the National Commission on Marihuana and Drug Abuse. Marihuana, A Signal of Misunderstanding, Commissioned by President Richard M. Nixon, March, 1972. Schaffer Library of Drug Policy. http://druglibrary.net/schaffer/Library/studies/nc/ncmenu.htm. Accessed October 22, 2018.

59   Young FL. Marijuana Rescheduling Petition - DEA, 1988. Schaffer Drug Library. http://www.druglibrary.org/schaffer/Library/studies/YOUNG/young4.html. Published September 6, 1988. Accessed July 4, 2018.

60   Rough L. A Guide to Federal Drug Rescheduling (And What It Means for Cannabis). Leafly. https://www.leafly.com/news/cannabis-101/a-guide-to-Federal-

drug-rescheduling-and-what-it-means-for-cannabis. Published July 9, 2018. Accessed October 22, 2018.

61   Marshall DR. Notice of Denial of Petition. US Department of Justice, DEA, Diversion Control Division. https://www.deadiversion.usdoj.gov/fed_regs/notices/2001/fr0418/fr0418a.htm. Published March 28, 2001. Accessed July 4, 2018.

62   The DEA Position on Marijuana. Drug Enforcement Administration. https://www.dea.gov/docs/marijuana_position_2011.pdf. Published April 2013. Accessed July 4, 2018.

63   Leonhart MM. Scheduling Review and Response to the Petition from the Coalition for Rescheduling Cannabis. US Department of Justice, DEA, Diversion Control Division. June 2011. https://www.deadiversion.usdoj.gov/pubs/coalition_response.pdf. Accessed July 4, 2018.

64   DeSalvo KB. DHHS Letter to Chuck Rosenberg. US Department of Justice, DEA, Diversion Control Division. June 2015. https://www.deadiversion.usdoj.gov/schedules/marijuana/Incoming_Letter_Department_HHS.pdf. Accessed July 5, 2018.

65   Drug Enforcement Administration, Rosenberg C. Office of the Federal Register. National Archives and Records Administration; 2016. https://www.federalregister.gov/documents/2016/08/12/2016-17954/denial-of-petition-to-initiate-proceedings-to-reschedule-marijuana. Accessed July 5, 2018.

66   Drug Enforcement Administration, Rosenberg C. Office of the Federal Register. National Archives and Records Administration; 2016. https://www.Federalregister.gov/documents/2016/08/12/2016-17960/denial-of-petition-to-initiate-proceedings-to-reschedule-marijuana. Accessed July 5, 2018.

67   Garvey T, Yeh BT. State Legalization of Recreational Marijuana: Selected Legal Issues.; 2014:10. https://fas.org/sgp/crs/misc/R43034.pdf. Accessed July 5, 2018.

68   Garvey T, Yeh BT. State Legalization of Recreational Marijuana: Selected Legal Issues.; 2014:11-12. https://fas.org/sgp/crs/misc/R43034.pdf. Accessed July 5, 2018.

69   Gonzales v. Raich. Oyez. https://www.oyez.org/cases/2004/03-1454. Published June 6, 2005. Accessed July 5, 2018.

70   Gonzales v. Raich. Oyez. https://www.oyez.org/cases/2004/03-1454. Published June 6, 2005. Accessed July 5, 2018.

71   Cambron C, Guttmannova K, Fleming CB. State and National Contexts in Evaluating Cannabis Laws: A Case Study of Washington State. Journal of drug issues. 2017;47(1):74-90. doi:10.1177/0022042616678607.

72   Deputy Attorney General, Cole JM. Memorandum For All United States Attorneys.
        https://www.justice.gov/iso/opa/resources/3052013829132756857467.pdf

73   Cambron C, Guttmannova K, Fleming CB. Journal of drug issues. https://www.ncbi.nlm.nih.gov/pmc/articles/PMC5404705/. Published January 2017. Accessed October 22, 2018.

74   Marijuana Enforcement . https://www.justice.gov/opa/press-release/file/1022196/download. Accessed December 6, 2018.

75   Justice Department Issues Memo on Marijuana Enforcement. The United States Department of Justice. https://www.justice.gov/opa/pr/justice-department-issues-memo-marijuana-enforcement. Published January 4, 2018. Accessed October 22, 2018.

76   FindLaw's United States Ninth Circuit case and opinions. Findlaw. https://caselaw.findlaw.com/us-9th-circuit/1253723.html. Accessed November 8, 2018.

77   Sec. 7606 the Legitimacy of Industrial Hemp Research of the Conference Report to accompany H.R. 2642. https://www.votehemp.com/wp-content/uploads/2018/07/Pages_from_farm0127.pdf Accessed December 6, 2018.

78   Establishment of a New Drug Code for Marihuana Extract A Rule by the Drug Enforcement Administration on 12/14/2016. Drug Enforcement Administration, Department of Justice. https://www.federalregister.gov/documents/2016/12/14/2016-29941/establishment-of-a-new-drug-code-for-marihuana-extract Accessed December 6, 2018

79   Molyneux RJ, Lee ST, Gardner DR, Panter KE, James LF. Phytochemicals: the good, the bad and the ugly. Phytochemistry. 2007;68(22–24):2973–85.

80   Harborne JB, Baxter H, Moss GP, eds. General Introduction. Phytochemical dictionary: a handbook of bioactive compounds from plants (2nd ed.). London: Taylor & Francis. 1999;vii.

81   "Phytochemicals". Micronutrient Information Center, Linus Pauling Institute, Oregon State University, Corvallis, OR. February 2016. https://lpi.oregonstate.edu/mic. Accessed December 8, 2018.

82   II. What we need to eat. Introduction to Nutrition -- Nutrients essential for man. https://library.med.utah.edu/NetBiochem/nutrition/lect1/2_4.html. Accessed October 22, 2018.

83   ElSohly MA. Marijuana and the Cannabinoids. Totowa, NJ: Humana Press; 2010.

84   Callaway JC. Hempseed as a nutritional resource: An overview. Euphytica. 2004;140, 65–72.

85   HEMP SEED: The Most Nutritionally Complete Food Source In The World. https://ratical.org/renewables/hempseed1.html. Accessed October 22, 2018.

86   ElSohly MA. Marijuana and the Cannabinoids. Totowa, NJ: Humana Press; 2010.
      http://www.medicinalgenomics.com/wp-content/uploads/2011/12/Chemical-constituents-of-cannabis.pdf. Accessed December 6, 2018.

87   Saxena M, Saxena J, Nema R, Singh D, Gupta A. Phytochemistry of Medicinal Plants. Journal of Pharmacognosy and Phytochemistry. 2013;1(6). http://www.phytojournal.com/vol1Issue6/26.html. Accessed December 8, 2018.

88   Fride E, Mechoulam R. Pharmacological activity of the cannabinoid receptor agonist, anandamide, a brain constituent. Eur J Pharmacol 1993;231(2):313–

4.

89   Malfait AM, Gallily R, Sumariwalla PF, Malik AS, Andreakos E, Mechoulam R, et al. The non-psychoactive cannabis constituent CBD is an oral anti-arthritic therapeutic in murine collagen-induced arthritis. Proc Natl Acad Sci USA 2000;97(17):9561–6.

90   Zuardi AW, Shirakawa I, Finkelfarb E, Karniol IG. Action of CBD on the anxiety and other effects produced by delta 9-THC in normal subjects. Psychopharmacology 1982;76(3):245–50.

91   Carlini EA, Cunha JM. Hypnotic and antiepileptic effects of CBD. J Clin Pharmacol 1981;21 (Suppl. 8–9):417S–27S.

92   Laprairie RB, Bagher AM, Kelly ME, Denovan-Wright EM Br J Pharmacol. 2015 Oct; 172(20):4790-805.

93   CBD displays unexpectedly high potency as an antagonist of CB1 and CB2 receptor agonists in vitro. *Thomas A, Baillie GL, Phillips AM, Razdan RK, Ross RA, Pertwee RG Br J Pharmacol. 2007 Mar; 150(5):613-23.*

94   McPartland JM, Russo EB. Cannabis and cannabis extracts: greater than the sum of their parts? Journal of Cannabis Therapeutics 2001;1(3–4):103–32.

95   Gertsch J. Anti-inflammatory cannabinoids in diet: towards a better understanding of CB(2) receptor action? Commun Integrative Biology. 2008;1:26-28

96   Martin S, Padilla E, Ocete M, Galvez J, Jiménez J, Zarzuelo A. "Anti-Inflammatory Activity of the Essential Oil of Bupleurum Fruticescens." Planta Med Planta Medica 59.06. 1993;533-36.

97   Tang H, Goldman D. Myocyte Enhancer Factor 2C (MEF-2C). Wiley Encyclopedia of Molecular Medicine. 2002; 372-78 doi:10.1002/0471203076. emm0743.

98   Appendino G, Gibbons S, Giana A, et al. Antibacterial Cannabinoids fromCannabis sativa: A Structure−Activity Study. Journal of Natural Products. 2008;71(8):1427-1430. doi:10.1021/np8002673.

99   Miyazawa M, Yamafuji C. Inhibition of Acetylcholinesterase Activity by Bicyclic Monoterpenoids. Journal of Agricultural and Food Chemistry. 2005;53(5):1765-1768. doi:10.1021/jf040019b.

100   Elisabetsky E, Marschner J, Souza DO. Effects of linalool on glutamatergic system in the rat cerebral cortex. Neurochemical Research. 1995;20(4):461-465. doi:10.1007/bf00973103.

101   Russo, Ethan. Handbook of Psychotropic Herbs: A Scientific Analysis of Herbal Remedies for Psychiatric Conditions. New York: Haworth Herbal, 2001.

102   Buchbauer G, Jirovetz L, Jäger W, Plank C, Dietrich H. Fragrance Compounds and Essential Oils with Sedative Effects upon Inhalation. Journal of Pharmaceutical Sciences. 1993;82(6):660-664. doi:10.1002/jps.2600820623.

103   Ghelardini C, Galeotti N, Salvatore G, Mazzanti G. Local Anaesthetic Activity of the Essential Oil of Lavandula angustifolia. Planta Medica. 1999;65(8):700-703. doi:10.1055/s-1999-14045.

104   Griesbach RJ. Biochemistry and Genetics of Flower Color. Plant Breeding Reviews. 2010:89-114. doi:10.1002/9780470650301.ch4.

105   Takahashi A, Ohnishi T. The Significance of the Study about the Biological Effects of Solar Ultraviolet Radiation using the Exposed Facility on the International Space Station. Biological Sciences in Space. 2004;18(4):255-260. doi:10.2187/bss.18.255.

106   Samanta A, Das G, Das S. Roles of flavonoids in plants. Int J Pharm Sci Tech. 2011;6, 12–35.

107   Kaul TN, Middleton E, Ogra PL. Antiviral effect of flavonoids on human viruses. Journal of Medical Virology. 1985;15(1):71-79. doi:10.1002/jmv.1890150110.

108   D-Alanine:D-alanine ligase as a new target for the flavonoids quercetin and apigenin. Wu D, Kong Y, Han C, Chen J, Hu L, Jiang H, Shen X Int J Antimicrob Agents. 2008 Nov; 32(5):421-6.

109   Madeswaran A, Umamaheswari M, Asokkumar K, Sivashanmugam T, Subhadradevi V, Jagannath P. Docking studies: In silico phosphodiesterase inhibitory activity of commercially available flavonoids. Bangladesh Journal of Pharmacology. 2012;7(1). doi:10.3329/bjp.v7i1.10595.

110   Paris D, Mathura V, Ait-Ghezala G, et al. Flavonoids lower Alzheimers Aß production via an NFkB dependent mechanism. Bioinformation. 2011;6(6):229-236. doi:10.6026/97320630006229.

111   Kerry NL, Abbey M. Red wine and fractionated phenolic compounds prepared from red wine inhibit low density lipoprotein oxidation in vitro1Supported by the National Heart Foundation of Australia and the Australian Atherosclerosis Society.1. Atherosclerosis. 1997;135(1):93-102. doi:10.1016/s0021-9150(97)00156-1.

112   Huang JH, Huang CC, Fang JY, Yang C, Chan CM, Wu NL, Kang SW, Hung CF. Protective effects of myricetin against ultraviolet-B-induced damage in human keratinocytes. Toxicol In Vitro. 2010 Feb; 24(1):21-8.

113   Hadi ME, Zhang F-J, Wu F-F, Zhou C-H, Tao J. Advances in Fruit Aroma Volatile Research. Molecules. 2013;18(7):8200-8229. doi:10.3390/molecules18078200.

114   Hadi ME, Zhang F-J, Wu F-F, Zhou C-H, Tao J. Advances in Fruit Aroma Volatile Research. Molecules. 2013;18(7):8200-8229. doi:10.3390/molecules18078200.

115   Clarke RC, Robert C, Merlin, ND. Cannabis: Evolution and Ethnobotany. Berkeley, California: University of California Press, 2013;26.

116   https://greensourcegardens.com/ Accessed December 6, 2018.

117   Granowicz J. The Endocannabinoid System: A History of Endocannabinoids and Cannabis. Marijuana Times Cannabis News. http://www.marijuanatimes.org/the-endocannabinoid-system-a-history-of-endocannabinoids-and-cannabis/. Published March 15, 2016. Accessed November 8, 2018.

118   Mcpartland JM, Matias I, Marzo VD, Glass M. Evolutionary origins of the

endocannabinoid system. Gene. 2006;370:64-74. doi:10.1016/j.gene.2005.11.004.

119   Aggarwal S. 'Tis in our nature: taking the human-cannabis relationship seriously in health science and public policy. Front Psychiatry. 2013;4:6. Published 2013 Feb 26. doi:10.3389/fpsyt.2013.00006

120   Alger B. Getting high on the endocannabinoid system. Cerebrum. 2013;2013:14. Published 2013 Nov 1.

121   Zou S, Kumar U. Cannabinoid Receptors and the Endocannabinoid System: Signaling and Function in the Central Nervous System. Int J Mol Sci. 2018;19(3):833. Published 2018 Mar 13. doi:10.3390/ijms19030833

122   The Science of the Endocannabinoid System: How THC Affects the Brain and the Body. The Science of Marijuana: How THC Affects the Brain | Scholastic: Nida. http://headsup.scholastic.com/students/endocannabinoid. Published 2011. Accessed November 12, 2018.

123   Pertwee RG. Cannabis and cannabinoids: pharmacology and rationale for clinical use. Pharm Sci 1997;3:539–45.

124   O'Sullivan SE. An update on peroxisome proliferator-activated receptor (PPAR) activation by cannabinoids. Br J Pharmacol. 2016;173:1899. [PMC free article] [PubMed]

125   Xiong W, Cheng K, Cui T, Godlewski G, Rice KC, Xu Y, Zhang L Nat Chem Biol. 2011 May;7(5):296-303.

126   Morales P, Hurst DP, Reggio PH. Molecular Targets of the Phytocannabinoids-A Complex Picture. Progress in the chemistry of organic natural products. 2017;103:103-131. doi:10.1007/978-3-319-45541-9_4.

127   Alban D. Anandamide: Putting The Bliss Molecule To Work For Your Brain. Reset.me. http://reset.me/story/anandamide-putting-the-bliss-molecule-to-work-for-your-brain/. Published March 29, 2016. Accessed November 12, 2018.

128   Deutsch DG, Ueda N, Yamamoto S. The fatty acid amide hydrolase (FAAH). Prostaglandins Leukot. Essent. Fat. Acids 2002;66, 201–210.

129   Dinh TP, Carpenter D, Leslie FM, et al. Brain monoglyceride lipase participating in endocannabinoid inactivation. Proc Natl Acad Sci U S A. 2002;99(16):10819-24.

130   Ahn K, McKinney MK, Cravatt BF. Enzymatic pathways that regulate endocannabinoid signaling in the nervous system. Chem Rev. 2008;108(5):1687-707.

131   Alger B. Getting high on the endocannabinoid system. Cerebrum. 2013;2013:14. Published 2013 Nov 1.

132   Drug Scheduling. DEA. https://www.dea.gov/druginfo/ds.shtml. Accessed November 12, 2018.

133   National Academies of Sciences, Engineering, and Medicine. 2017. The Health Effects of Cannabis and Cannabinoids: The Current State of Evidence and Recommendations for Research. Washington, DC: The National Academies Press. https://doi.org/10.17226/24625.

134   National Institute on Drug Abuse. Opioid Overdose Crisis. NIDA. https://www.drugabuse.gov/drugs-abuse/opioids/opioid-crisis. Published March 6, 2018. Accessed November 12, 2018.

135   Bachhuber MA, Saloner B, Cunningham CO, Barry CL. Medical Cannabis Laws and Opioid Analgesic Overdose Mortality in the United States, 1999-2010. JAMA Intern Med. 2014;174(10):1668–1673. doi:10.1001/jamainternmed.2014.4005

136   Shi Y. Medical marijuana policies and hospitalizations related to marijuana and opioid pain reliever. Current neurology and neuroscience reports. https://www.ncbi.nlm.nih.gov/pubmed/28259087. Published April 1, 2017. Accessed November 13, 2018.

137   Shi Y. Medical marijuana policies and hospitalizations related to marijuana and opioid pain reliever. Current neurology and neuroscience reports. https://www.ncbi.nlm.nih.gov/pubmed/28259087. Published April 1, 2017. Accessed November 13, 2018.

138   Grant I, Cahn BR. Cannabis and endocannabinoid modulators: Therapeutic promises and challenges. Clinical neuroscience research. 2005;5(2-4):185-199. doi:10.1016/j.cnr.2005.08.015

139   Manzanares, J., Julian, M., & Carrascosa, A. (2006). Role of the Cannabinoid System in Pain Control and Therapeutic Implications for the Management of Acute and Chronic Pain Episodes. Current Neuropharmacology. 2006;4(3):239–257.

140   Manzanares J, Julian M, Carrascosa A. Role of the Cannabinoid System in Pain Control and Therapeutic Implications for the Management of Acute and Chronic Pain Episodes. Current Neuropharmacology. 2006;4(3):239–257.

141   Manzanares J, Julian M, Carrascosa A. Role of the Cannabinoid System in Pain Control and Therapeutic Implications for the Management of Acute and Chronic Pain Episodes. Current Neuropharmacology. 2006;4(3):239–257.

142   Manzanares J, Julian M, Carrascosa A. Role of the Cannabinoid System in Pain Control and Therapeutic Implications for the Management of Acute and Chronic Pain Episodes. Current Neuropharmacology. 2006;4(3):239–257.

143   Small-Howard AL, Shimoda LM, Adra CN, Turner H. Anti-inflammatory potential of CB1-mediated cAMP elevation in mast cells. Current neurology and neuroscience reports. https://www.ncbi.nlm.nih.gov/pubmed/15669919. Published June 1, 2005. Accessed November 13, 2018.

144   Andrews PLR, Horn CC. Signals for nausea and emesis: Implications for models of upper gastrointestinal diseases. *Autonomic neuroscience : basic & clinical.* 2006;125(1-2):100-115.
       doi:10.1016/j.autneu.2006.01.008.

145   Badowski ME. A review of oral cannabinoids and medical marijuana for the treatment of chemotherapy-induced nausea and vomiting: a focus on pharmacokinetic variability and pharmacodynamics. Current neurology and neuroscience reports. https://www.ncbi.nlm.nih.gov/pubmed/28780725.   Published   September   2017. Accessed November 13, 2018.

146   Matsumaru A, Tsutsumi Y, Ito S. Comparative investigation of the anti-emetic effects of granisetron and palonosetron during the treatment of acute

myeloid leukemia. Molecular and Clinical Oncology, 2017;7(4): 629–632. http://doi.org/10.3892/mco.2017.1350

147   Vazin A, Eslami D, Sahebi E. Evaluating the antiemetic administration consistency to prevent chemotherapy-induced nausea and vomiting with the standard guidelines: a prospective observational study. Therapeutics and Clinical Risk Management, 2017;13:1151–1157. http://doi.org/10.2147/TCRM.S133820

148   Rudd JA, Andrews PL. Mechanisms of acute, delayed and anticipatory emesis induced by anticancer therapies. In: Hesketh PJ, editor. Management of nausea and vomiting in cancer and cancer treatment. Sudbury, MA: Jones and Bartlett Publishers; 2005:15–66.

149   Hesketh PJ, Bohlke K, Lyman GH, et al. Antiemetics: American Society of Clinical Oncology focused guideline update. J Clin Oncol. 2016;34(4):381–386.

150   Saito R, Takano Y, Kamiya HO. Roles of substance P and NK(1) receptor in the brainstem in the development of emesis. J Pharmacol Sci. 2003;91(2):87–94.

151   The Antiemetic Subcommittee of the Multinational Association of Supportive Care in Cancer (MASCC); Prevention of chemotherapy- and radiotherapy-induced emesis: results of the 2004 Perugia International Antiemetic Consensus Conference, *Annals of Oncology*, 2005;17(1):20-28. https://doi.org/10.1093/annonc/mdj078

152   https://www.accessdata.fda.gov/drugsatfda_docs/label/2017/018651s029lbl.pdf Accessed December 6, 2018

153   https://www.accessdata.fda.gov/drugsatfda_docs/label/2006/018677s011lbl.pdf Accessed December6, 2018

154   Cotter J. Efficacy of Crude Marijuana and Synthetic Delta-9-Tetrahydrocannabinol as Treatment for Chemotherapy-Induced Nausea and Vomiting: A Systematic Literature Review. Oncol Nurs Forum. 2009;36(3):345-352.

155   Parker LA, Rock EM, Limebeer CL. Regulation of nausea and vomiting by cannabinoids. British Journal of Pharmacology. 2011;163(7):1411-1422. doi:10.1111/j.1476-5381.2010.01176.x.

156   Van Sickle MD, Oland LD, Ho W, et al. Cannabinoids inhibit emesis through CB1 receptors in the brainstem of the ferret. Gastroenterology. 2000;121(4):767-74.

157   Parker LA, Rock EM, Limebeer CL. Regulation of nausea and vomiting by cannabinoids. British Journal of Pharmacology. 2011;163(7):1411-1422. doi:10.1111/j.1476-5381.2010.01176.x.

158   Rock EM, Connolly C, Limebeer CL, et al. Psychopharmacology. 2016;233(18):3353-3360. https://doi.org/10.1007/s00213-016-4378-7

159   Tramèr MR, Carroll D, Campbell FA, et al. Cannabinoids for control of chemotherapy induced nausea and vomiting: quantitative systematic review. BMJ : British Medical Journal. 2001;323(7303):16.

160   Hugos CL, Bourdette D, Chen Y, et al. A group-delivered self-management program reduces spasticity in people with multiple sclerosis: A randomized, controlled pilot trial. Multiple Sclerosis Journal - Experimental, Translational and Clinical. 2017;3(1). http://doi.org/10.1177/2055217317699993

161   Beard S, Hunn A, Wight J. Treatments for spasticity and pain in multiple sclerosis: a systematic review. Health Technol Assess. 2003;7(40).

162   Sativex Oromucosal Spray. Glyceryl Trinitrate Tablets 500 micrograms - Summary of Product Characteristics (SmPC) - (eMC). https://www.medicines.org.uk/ emc/product/602/smpc#PHARMACOLOGICAL_PROPS. Published June 16, 2010. Accessed November 24, 2018.

163   Mecha M, Feliú A, Iñigo PM, et al. Cannabidiol Provides Long-lasting Protection Against the Deleterious Effects of Inflammation in a Viral Model of Multiple Sclerosis: A Role for A2A Receptor. Neurobiology of Disease. 2013;59:141-150. ISSN 0969-9961, https://doi.org/10.1016/j.nbd.2013.06.016.

164   Giacoppo S, Pollastro F, Grassi G, Bramanti P, Mazzon E. Target Regulation of PI3K/Akt/mTOR Pathway by Cannabidiol in Treatment of Experimental Multiple Sclerosis. Fitoterapia. 2017;116:77-84. ISSN 0367-326X, https://doi.org/10.1016/j. fitote.2016.11.010.

165   Giacoppo S, Pollastro F, Grassi G, Bramanti P, Mazzon E. Target Regulation of PI3K/Akt/mTOR Pathway by Cannabidiol in Treatment of Experimental Multiple Sclerosis. Fitoterapia. 2017;116:77-84. ISSN 0367-326X, https://doi.org/10.1016/j. fitote.2016.11.010.

166   Zajicek, John et al. Cannabinoids for Treatment of Spasticity and Other Symptoms Related to Multiple Sclerosis (CAMS study): Multicentre Randomised Placebo-controlled Trial. The Lancet. 2003;362(9395): 1517-1526.

167   Chong M S, Wolff K, et al. Cannabis Use in Patients with Multiple Sclerosis. Multiple Sclerosis Journal. 2006;12(5):646-651. Doi: 10.1177/1352458506070947

168   Badowski, M. E., & Perez, S. E. (2016). Clinical utility of dronabinol in the treatment of weight loss associated with HIV and AIDS. HIV/AIDS (Auckland, N.Z.), 8, 37–45. http://doi.org/10.2147/HIV.S81420

169   Badowski, M. E., & Perez, S. E. (2016). Clinical utility of dronabinol in the treatment of weight loss associated with HIV and AIDS. HIV/AIDS (Auckland, N.Z.), 8, 37–45. http://doi.org/10.2147/HIV.S81420

170   Marinol (dronabinol) [package insert] North Chicago, IL: AbbVie, Inc.; 2013.

171   Hengge UR, Stocks K, Wiehler H, et al. Double-blind, randomized, placebo-controlled phase III trial of oxymetholone for the treatment of HIV wasting. AIDS. 2003;17:699–710.

172   Kaplan G, Thomas S, Fierer DS, et al. Thalidomide for the treatment of AIDS-associated wasting. AIDS Res Hum Retroviruses. 2000;16:1345–1355.

173   Megace (megestrol acetate, USP) Oral Suspension [Package Insert]. (2016). Princeton, New Jersey: Bristol-Meyers Squibb Company.

174   Remeron (mirtazapine) [package insert] White Station, NJ: Merck and Co., Inc.; 2011.

175   Marinol (dronabinol) [package insert] North Chicago, IL: AbbVie, Inc.; 2013.

176   Beal JE, Olson R, Lefkowitz L, Laubenstein L, Bellman P, Yangco B, Morales JO, Murphy R, Powderly W, Plasse TF, Mosdell KW, Shepard KV. Long-term efficacy and safety of dronabinol for acquired immunodeficiency syndrome-associated anorexia. J Pain Symptom Manage. 1997l;14(1):7-14. DOI: 10.1016/S0885-3924(97)00038-9

177   Williams CM, Rogers PJ, Kirkham TC. Hyperphagia in pre-fed rats following oral delta9-THC. Physiol Behav. 1998;65(2):343-6. DOI: 10.1016/S0031-9384(98)00170-X.

178   Berry Elliot M, Mechoulam Raphael. Tetrahydrocannabinol and endocannabinoids in feeding and appetite. Pharmacology & Therapeutics. 2002;95(2):185-190. DOI:10.1016/S0163-7258(02)00257-7.

179   Beal JE, Olson R, Laubenstein L, et al. Dronabinol as a treatment for anorexia associated with weight loss in patients with AIDS.J Pain Symptom Manage. 1995;10(2):89-97.

180   Plasse TF, Gorter RW, Krasnow SH, et al. Recent clinical experience with dronabinol. Pharmacol Biochem Behav. 1991;40(3):695-700. DOI: 10.1016/0091-3057(91)90385-F

181   Riggs Patricia K, Vaida Florin, Rossi Steven S, et al. A pilot study of the effects of cannabis on appetite hormones in HIV-infected adult men. Brain Research. 2012;1431:46-52. DOI:10.1016/j.brainres.2011.11.001.

182   Roessner V, Plessen KJ, Rothenberger A, et al. The ESSTS Guidelines Group. European clinical guidelines for Tourette syndrome and other tic disorders. Part II: pharmacological treatment. European Child & Adolescent Psychiatry. 2011;20(4):173–196. http://doi.org/10.1007/s00787-011-0163-7

183   Müller-Vahl KR, Schneider U, Koblenz A, et al. Treatment of Tourette's Syndrome with □⁹-Tetrahydrocannabinol (THC): A Randomized Crossover Trial. Pharmacopsychiatry. 2002;35(2):57-61. DOI: 10.1055/s-2002-25028

184   Abi-Jaoude E, Chen L, Cheung P, Bhikram T, Sandor P. Preliminary Evidence on Cannabis Effectiveness and Tolerability for Adults With Tourette Syndrome. J Neuropsychiatry Clin Neurosci. 2017;29(4):391-400. DOI: 10.1176/appi.neuropsych.16110310.

185   American Psychiatric Association. Diagnostic and statistical manual of mental disorders: DSM-5(5th ed.) American Psychiatric Association. 2013;5:222-226.

186   Practice Guideline for the Treatment of Patients With Panic Disorder. https://psychiatryonline.org/pb/assets/raw/sitewide/practice_guidelines/guidelines/panicdisorder.pdf. Accessed 10 Aug. 2018.

187   Hernandez I, He M, Brooks MM, Zhang Y. Exposure-Response Association Between Concurrent Opioid and Benzodiazepine Use and Risk of Opioid-Related Overdose in Medicare Part D Beneficiaries. JAMA Network Open. 2018;1(2):e180919. doi:10.1001/jamanetworkopen.2018.0919

188   Schier, Alexandre Rafael de Mello, Ribeiro, Natalia Pinho de Oliveira, Silva, Adriana Cardoso de Oliveira e, Hallak, Jaime Eduardo Cecílio, Crippa, José Alexandre S., Nardi, Antonio E., & Zuardi, Antonio Waldo. (2012). Cannabidiol, a Cannabis sativa constituent, as an anxiolytic drug. Revista Brasileira de Psiquiatria,

34(Suppl. 1), 104-110. https://dx.doi.org/10.1590/S1516-44462012000500008

189   Resstel LB, Tavares RF, Lisboa SF, Joca SR, Corrêa FM, Guimarães FS. 5-HT1A receptors are involved in the cannabidiol-induced attenuation of behavioural and cardiovascular responses to acute restraint stress in rats. British Journal of Pharmacology. 2009;156(1):181-188. doi:10.1111/j.1476-5381.2008.00046.x.

190   Resstel LB, Tavares RF, Lisboa SF, Joca SR, Corrêa FM, Guimarães FS. 5-HT1A receptors are involved in the cannabidiol-induced attenuation of behavioural and cardiovascular responses to acute restraint stress in rats. British Journal of Pharmacology. 2009;156(1):181-188. doi:10.1111/j.1476-5381.2008.00046.x.

191   Rock EM, Limebeer CL, Petric GN, Wiliams LA, Mechoulam R, Parker LA. Effect of prior foot shock stress and Δ9-tetrahydrocannabinol, cannabidiolic acid, and cannabidiol on anxiety-like responding in the light-dark emergence test in rats. Psychopharmacology (Berl). 2017 Jul;234(14):2207-2215. DOI: 10.1007/s00213-01704626-5.

192   Schier, Alexandre Rafael de Mello, Ribeiro, Natalia Pinho de Oliveira, Silva, Adriana Cardoso de Oliveira e, Hallak, Jaime Eduardo Cecílio, Crippa, José Alexandre S., Nardi, Antonio E., & Zuardi, Antonio Waldo. (2012). Cannabidiol, a Cannabis sativa constituent, as an anxiolytic drug. Revista Brasileira de Psiquiatria, 34(Suppl. 1), 104-110. https://dx.doi.org/10.1590/S1516-44462012000500008

193   Schier, Alexandre Rafael de Mello, Ribeiro, Natalia Pinho de Oliveira, Silva, Adriana Cardoso de Oliveira e, Hallak, Jaime Eduardo Cecílio, Crippa, José Alexandre S., Nardi, Antonio E., & Zuardi, Antonio Waldo. (2012). Cannabidiol, a Cannabis sativa constituent, as an anxiolytic drug. Revista Brasileira de Psiquiatria, 34(Suppl. 1), 104-110. https://dx.doi.org/10.1590/S1516-44462012000500008

194   American Psychiatric Association. (2013). Diagnostic and statistical manual of mental disorders: DSM-5(5th ed.). 271-280. Arlington, VA: American Psychiatric Association.

195   "Treatment of PTSD - PTSD: National Center ...." 18 Aug. 2017, https://www.ptsd.va.gov/public/treatment/therapy-med/treatment-ptsd.asp. Accessed 7 Aug. 2018.

196   "PTSD - American Psychological Association." https://www.apa.org/ptsd-guideline/ptsd.pdf. Accessed 9 Aug. 2018.

197   Jetly R, Heber A, Fraser G, Boisvert D. The Efficacy of Nabilone, a synthetic cannabinoid, in the treatment of PTSD-associated Nightmares: A Preliminary Randomized, Double-Blind, Placebo-controlled Cross-over Design Study. Psychoneuroendocrinology. 2015 Jan; 51:585-8. Doi: 10.106/j.psyneuen.2014.11.002#

198   Gentes EL, Schry AR, Hicks TA, et al. Prevalence and Correlates of Cannabis Use in an Outpatient VA Posttraumatic Stress Disorder Clinic. Psychology of addictive behaviors : journal of the Society of Psychologists in Addictive Behaviors. 2016;30(3):415-421. doi:10.1037/adb0000154.

199   Manhapra A, Stefanovics E, Rosenheck R. Treatment outcomes for veterans with PTSD and substance use: Impact of specific substances and achievement of abstinence. Drug and alcohol dependence. 2015;156:70-77. doi:10.1016/j.drugalcdep.2015.08.036.

200   National Eye Institute. "Facts about Glaucoma". https://nei.nih.gov/health/

glaucoma/glaucoma_facts. Accessed 21 June 2018.

201   "Xalatan (latanoprost) Ophthalmic Solution, Labeling Revision - FDA."
https://www.accessdata.fda.gov/drugsatfda_docs/label/2012/020597s044lbl.pdf.
Accessed 9 Aug. 2018.

202   "TIMOPTIC-XE® 0.25% and 0.5% (TIMOLOL MALEATE ... - FDA."
https://www.accessdata.fda.gov/drugsatfda_docs/label/2015/020330s029lbl.pdf.
Accessed 9 Aug. 2018.

203   El-Remessy AB, Khalil IE, Matragoon S, et al. Neuroprotective Effect
of(−)Δ9-Tetrahydrocannabinol and Cannabidiol in N-Methyl-d-Aspartate-Induced
Retinal Neurotoxicity : Involvement of Peroxynitrite. The American Journal of
Pathology. 2003;163(5):1997-2008.

204   Hampson AJ, Grimaldi M, Axelrod J, Wink D. Cannabidiol and (−)Δ9-
tetrahydrocannabinol are neuroprotective antioxidants. Proceedings of the National
Academy of Sciences of the United States of America. 1998;95(14):8268-8273.

205   El-Remessy AB, Khalil IE, Matragoon S, et al. Neuroprotective Effect
of(−)Δ9-Tetrahydrocannabinol and Cannabidiol in N-Methyl-d-Aspartate-Induced
Retinal Neurotoxicity : Involvement of Peroxynitrite. The American Journal of
Pathology. 2003;163(5):1997-2008.

206   Yazulla S, Studholme KM, McIntosh HH, Deutsch DG:
Immunocytochemical localization of cannabinoid CB1 receptor and fatty acid amide
hydrolase in rat retina. J Comp Neurol 1999, 415:80-90

207   El-Remessy AB, Khalil IE, Matragoon S, et al. Neuroprotective Effect
of(−)Δ9-Tetrahydrocannabinol and Cannabidiol in N-Methyl-d-Aspartate-Induced
Retinal Neurotoxicity : Involvement of Peroxynitrite. The American Journal of
Pathology. 2003;163(5):1997-2008.

208   Tomida I, Azuara-Blanco A, House H, Flint M, Pertwee RG, Robson PJ.
Effect of Sublingual Application of Cannabinoids on Intraocular Pressure: A Pilot
Study. J Glaucoma. 2006 Oct; 15(5):349-53.

209   "American Academy of Ophthalmology Reiterates Position that ...."
Accessed July 23, 2018. https://www.aao.org/newsroom/news-releases/detail/
american-academy-of-ophthalmology-reiterates-posit.

210   Pawlotsky JM. Hepatitis C virus: standard-of-care treatment. Adv
Pharmacol. 2013;67:169-215. DOI: 10.1016/B978-0-12-405880-4.00005-6.

211   "PEG-Intron (Peginterferon alfa-2b) Package Insert - FDA." https://www.
accessdata.fda.gov/drugsatfda_docs/label/2001/pegsche080701LB.htm. Accessed 19
Aug. 2018.

212   "Rebetol (ribavirin) Package Insert - FDA." https://www.accessdata.fda.
gov/drugsatfda_docs/label/2007/020903s040lbl.pdf. Accessed 19 Aug. 2018.

213   Pawlotsky JM. Hepatitis C virus: standard-of-care treatment. Adv
Pharmacol. 2013;67:169-215. DOI: 10.1016/B978-0-12-405880-4.00005-6.

214   "Direct-acting antivirals for the treatment of hepatitis C virus infection
...." 24 Aug. 2017, https://www.uptodate.com/contents/direct-acting-antivirals-for-
the-treatment-of-hepatitis-c-virus-infection. Accessed 19 Aug. 2018.

215   "Will Hepatitis C Virus Medication Costs Drop in the Years Ahead?." 8 Feb. 2017, https://www.pharmacytimes.com/resource-centers/hepatitisc/will-hepatitis-c-virus-medicaton-costs-drop-in-the-years-ahead. Accessed 19 Aug. 2018.

216   Lowe HIC, Toyang NJ, McLaughlin W. Potential of Cannabidiol for the Treatment of Viral Hepatitis. Pharmacognosy Research. 2017;9(1):116-118. DOI:10.4103/0974-8490.199780.

217   Sylvestre DL1, Clements BJ, Malibu Y. Cannabis use improves retention and virological outcomes in patients treated for hepatitis C. Eur J Gastroenterol Hepatol. 2006 Oct;18(10):1057-63. DOI:
       10.1097/01.meg.0000216934.22114.51.

218   "Rebetol (ribavirin) Package Insert - FDA." https://www.accessdata.fda.gov/drugsatfda_docs/label/2007/020903s040lbl.pdf. Accessed 19 Aug. 2018.

219   "PEG-Intron (Peginterferon alfa-2b) Package Insert - FDA." https://www.accessdata.fda.gov/drugsatfda_docs/label/2001/pegsche080701LB.htm. Accessed 19 Aug. 2018.

220   Teixeira-Clerc F, Julien B, Grenard P, Tran Van Nhieu J, Deveaux V, Li L, Serriere-Lanneau V, Ledent C, Mallat A, Lotersztajn S. CB1 cannabinoid receptor antagonism: a new strategy for the treatment of liver fibrosis. *Nat Med.* 2006 Jun;12(6):671-6. Epub 2006 May 21. DOI: 10.1038/nm1421

221   Julien Boris, Pascale Grenard, Teixeira-Clerc Fatima, Tran Van Nhieu Jeanne, Li Liying, Karsak Meliha, Zimmer Andreas, Mallat Ariane, Lotersztajn Sophie. Antifibrogenic role of the cannabinoid receptor CB2 in the liver. Gastroenterology. 2005. 128(3):742-55. DOI: 10.1053/j.gastro.2004.12.050

222   Ishida JH, Peters MG, Jin C, et al. Influence of Cannabis Use on Severity of Hepatitis C Disease. Clinical gastroenterology and hepatology : the official clinical practice journal of the American Gastroenterological Association. 2008;6(1):69-75. doi:10.1016/j.cgh.2007.10.021.

223   Tortarolo M, Lo Coco D, Veglianese P, et al. Amyotrophic Lateral Sclerosis, a Multisystem Pathology: Insights into the Role of TNFα. Mediators of Inflammation. 2017;2017:2985051. doi:10.1155/2017/2985051.

224   "RILUTEK® (riluzole) Tablets Rx only DESCRIPTION RILUTEK ... - FDA." https://www.accessdata.fda.gov/drugsatfda_docs/label/2009/020599s011s012lbl.pdf. Accessed 9 Aug. 2018.

225   Carter GT, Abood ME, Aggarwal SK, Weiss MD. Cannabis and amyotrophic lateral sclerosis: hypothetical and practical applications, and a call for clinical trials. Am J Hosp Palliat Care. 2010 Aug;27(5):347-56. DOI: 10.1177/1049909110369531.

226   Silvia Rossi, Valentina De Chiara, Alessandra Musella, Mauro Cozzolino, Giorgio Bernardi, Mauro Maccarrone, Nicola B. Mercuri, Maria Teresa Carrì & Diego Centonze (2010) Abnormal sensitivity of cannabinoid CB1 receptors in the striatum of mice with experimental amyotrophic lateral sclerosis, Amyotrophic Lateral Sclerosis, 11:1-2, 83-90, DOI: 10.3109/17482960902977954

227   Bilsland LG, Dick JR, Pryce G, Petrosino S, Di Marzo V, Baker D, Greensmith L. Increasing cannabinoid levels by pharmacological and genetic manipulation delay disease progression in SOD1 mice. FASE J. 2006 May; 20(7):1003-

5. DOI: 10.1096/fj.05-4743fje

228   Yiangou Y, Facer P, Durrenberger P, et al. COX-2, CB2 and P2X7-immunoreactivities are increased in activated microglial cells/macrophages of multiple sclerosis and amyotrophic lateral sclerosis spinal cord. BMC Neurology. 2006;6:12. doi:10.1186/1471-2377-6-12.

229   Carter GT, Abood ME, Aggarwal SK, Weiss MD. Cannabis and amyotrophic lateral sclerosis: hypothetical and practical applications, and a call for clinical trials. Am J Hosp Palliat Care. 2010 Aug;27(5):347-56. DOI: 10.1177/1049909110369531.

230   Carter GT, Abood ME, Aggarwal SK, Weiss MD. Cannabis and amyotrophic lateral sclerosis: hypothetical and practical applications, and a call for clinical trials. Am J Hosp Palliat Care. 2010 Aug;27(5):347-56. DOI: 10.1177/1049909110369531.

231   Lichtenstein GR, Loftus EV, Isaacs KL, Regueiro MD, Gerson LB, Sands BE. ACG Clinical Guideline: Management of Crohn's Disease in Adults. Am J Gastroenterol. 2018 Apr;113(4):481-517. Epub 2018 Mar 27. DOI: 10.1038/ajg.2018.27.

232   Kuhbacher T, Fölsch U. Practical guidelines for the treatment of inflammatory bowel disease. World Journal of Gastroenterology : WJG. 2007;13(8):1149-1155. doi:10.3748/wjg.v13.i8.1149.

233   Kornbluth A, Sachar DB; Practice Parameters Committee of the American College of Gastroenterology.Ulcerative colitis practice guidelines in adults: American College Of Gastroenterology, Practice Parameters Committee. Am J Gastroenterol. 2010 Mar;105(3):501-23. Epub 2010 Jan 12. DOI: 10.1038/ajg.2009.727.

234   "Azulfidine EN-tabs® sulfasalazine delayed release tablets, USP ... - FDA." https://www.accessdata.fda.gov/drugsatfda_docs/label/2012/007073s125lbl.pdf. Accessed 18 Aug. 2018.

235   O'Donnell S, O'Morain CA. Therapeutic benefits of budesonide in gastroenterology. Therapeutic Advances in Chronic Disease. 2010;1(4):177-186. doi:10.1177/2040622310379293.

236   "PRODUCT INFORMATION IMURAN (azathioprine) 50-mg ... - FDA." https://www.accessdata.fda.gov/drugsatfda_docs/label/2011/016324s034s035lbl.pdf. Accessed 18 Aug. 2018.

237   "REMICADE (infliximab) Label - FDA." https://www.accessdata.fda.gov/drugsatfda_docs/label/2013/103772s5359lbl.pdf. Accessed 18 Aug. 2018.

238   "Humira (adalimumab) label - FDA." https://www.accessdata.fda.gov/drugsatfda_docs/label/2011/125057s0276lbl.pdf. Accessed 18 Aug. 2018.

239   Hornby PJ, Prouty SM. Involvement of cannabinoid receptors in gut motility and visceral perception. British Journal of Pharmacology. 2004;141(8):1335-1345. doi:10.1038/sj.bjp.0705783.

240   Schicho R, Storr M. Cannabis finds its way into treatment of Crohn's disease. Pharmacology. 2014;93(0):1-3. doi:10.1159/000356512.

241   Hasenoehrl C, Taschler U, Storr M, Schicho R. The gastrointestinal tract – a central organ of cannabinoid signaling in health and disease. Neurogastroenterology and motility : the official journal of the European Gastrointestinal Motility Society.

2016;28(12):1765-1780. doi:10.1111/nmo.12931.

242 Marquéz L, Suárez J, Iglesias M, Bermudez-Silva FJ, Rodríguez de Fonseca F, Andreu M. Ulcerative Colitis Induces Changes on the Expression of the Endocannabinoid System in the Human Colonic Tissue. Bereswill S, ed. PLoS ONE. 2009;4(9):e6893. doi:10.1371/journal.pone.0006893.

243 Schicho R, Storr M. Cannabis finds its way into treatment of Crohn's disease. Pharmacology. 2014;93(0):1-3. doi:10.1159/000356512.

244 Schicho R, Storr M. Cannabis finds its way into treatment of Crohn's disease. Pharmacology. 2014;93(0):1-3. doi:10.1159/000356512.

245 Jamontt J, Molleman A, Pertwee R, Parsons M. The effects of Δ9-tetrahydrocannabinol and cannabidiol alone and in combination on damage, inflammation and in vitro motility disturbances in rat colitis. British Journal of Pharmacology. 2010;160(3):712-723. doi:10.1111/j.1476-5381.2010.00791.x.

246 American Psychiatric Association. (2013). Diagnostic and statistical manual of mental disorders : DSM-5(5th ed.). 611-614 Arlington, VA: American Psychiatric Association.

247 Geldmacher DS. Treatment Guidelines for Alzheimer's Disease: Redefining Perceptions in Primary Care. Primary Care Companion to The Journal of Clinical Psychiatry. 2007;9(2):113-121.

248 "Aricept (donepezil hydrochloride) Label - FDA." https://www.accessdata. fda.gov/drugsatfda_docs/label/2012/020690s035,021720s008,022568s005lbl.pdf. Accessed 17 Aug. 2018.

249 "Namenda (memantine hydrochloride) Label (PDF) - FDA." https://www. accessdata.fda.gov/drugsatfda_docs/label/2013/021487s010s012s014,021627s008lbl. pdf. Accessed 17 Aug. 2018.

250 Luvone T, Esposito G, Esposito R, Santamaria R, Di Rosa M, Izzo AA. Neuroprotective effect of cannabidiol, a non-psychoactive component from Cannabis sativa, on beta-amyloid-induced toxicity in PC12 cells. J Neurochem. 2004 Apr;89(1):134-41. DOI: 10.1111/j.1471-4159.2003.02327.x.

251 Stumm Christoph, Hiebel Christof, Hanstein Regina, Purrio Martin, Nagel Heike, Conrad Andrea, Lutz Beat, Behl Christian, Clement Angela. Cannabinoid receptor 1 deficiency in a mouse model of Alzheimer's disease leads to enhanced cognitive impairment despite of a reduction in amyloid deposition. Neurobiology of Aging. 2013 Nov. 34(11): 2574-2584.

252 Aso E, Ferrer I. Cannabinoids for treatment of Alzheimer's disease: moving toward the clinic. Frontiers in Pharmacology. 2014;5:37. doi:10.3389/fphar.2014.00037.

253 Volicer L, Stelly M, Morris J, McLaughlin J, Volicer BJ. Effects of dronabinol on anorexia and disturbed behavior in patients with Alzheimer's disease. Int J Geriatr Psychiatry. 1997 Sep;12(9):913-9.

254 Walther S, Mahlberg R, Eichmann U, Kunz D. Delta-9-tetrahydrocannabinol for nighttime agitation in severe dementia.Psychopharmacology (Berl). 2006 May;185(4):524-8. Epub 2006 Mar 7. DOI: 10.1007/s00213-006-0343-1.

255   Iring A, Ruisanchez É, Leszl-Ishiguro M, Horváth B, Benkő R, Lacza Z, Járai Z, Sándor P, Di Marzo V, Pacher P, Benyó Z.Role of endocannabinoids and cannabinoid-1 receptors in cerebrocortical blood flow regulation. PLoS One. 2013;8(1):e53390. Epub 2013 Jan 4. DOI: 10.1371/journal.pone.0053390.

256   "Epilepsy Foundation." https://www.epilepsy.com/. Accessed 18 Aug. 2018.

257   Fisher R. S., Boas W. V., Blume W. , Elger C. , Genton P., Lee P., and Engel J. Epileptic Seizures and Epilepsy: Definitions Proposed by the International League Against Epilepsy (ILAE) and the International Bureau for Epilepsy (IBE). Epilepsia, 2005. 46: 470-472. DOI:10.1111/j.0013-9580.2005.66104.x

258   Organización Mundial de la Salud. Programme for Neurological Diseases, et al. Atlas: epilepsy care in the world. World Health Organization, 2005.

259   Fisher R. S., Boas W. V., Blume W. , Elger C. , Genton P., Lee P., and Engel J. Epileptic Seizures and Epilepsy: Definitions Proposed by the International League Against Epilepsy (ILAE) and the International Bureau for Epilepsy (IBE). Epilepsia, 2005. 46: 470-472.

260   Fisher R. S., Cross J. H., French J. A., Higurashi N. , Hirsch E. , Jansen F. E., Lagae L. , Moshé S. L., Peltola J., Roulet Perez E., Scheffer I. E., and Zuberi, S. M. Operational classification of seizure types by the International League Against Epilepsy: Position Paper of the ILAE Commission for Classification and Terminology. Epilepsia, 2017.n58: 522-530. DOI:10.1111/epi.13670

261   Glauser T, Ben-Menachem E, Bourgeois B, Cnaan A, Chadwick D, Guerreiro C, Kalviainen R, Mattson R, Perucca E, Tomson, T. ILAE Treatment Guidelines: Evidence-based Analysis of Antiepileptic Drug Efficacy and Effectiveness as Initial Monotherapy for Epileptic Seizures and Syndromes. Epilepsia, 2006.47: 1094-1120. DOI:10.1111/j.1528-1167.2006.00585.x

262   "Tegretol® Tegretol®-XR WARNINGS - Novartis Pharmaceuticals ...." https://www.pharma.us.novartis.com/product/pi/pdf/tegretol.pdf. Accessed 18 Aug. 2018.

263   "Dilantin (phenytoin sodium) - FDA." https://www.accessdata.fda.gov/drugsatfda_docs/label/2009/084349s060lbl.pdf. Accessed 18 Aug. 2018.

264   "Mysoline® (primidone, USP) - FDA." https://www.accessdata.fda.gov/drugsatfda_docs/label/2009/009170s036lbl.pdf. Accessed 18 Aug. 2018.

265   "Depakote (divalproex sodium) Tablets - FDA." https://www.accessdata.fda.gov/drugsatfda_docs/label/2011/018723s037lbl.pdf. Accessed 18 Aug. 2018.

266   "Sabril (vigabatrin) - FDA." https://www.accessdata.fda.gov/drugsatfda_docs/label/2013/020427s010s011s012,022006s011s012s013lbl.pdf. Accessed 18 Aug. 2018.

267   "NEURONTIN (gabapentin) - FDA." https://www.accessdata.fda.gov/drugsatfda_docs/label/2017/020235s064_020882s047_021129s046lbl.pdf. Accessed 18 Aug. 2018.

268   "TRILEPTAL (oxcarbazepine) - FDA." https://www.accessdata.fda.gov/drugsatfda_docs/label/2017/021014s036lbl.pdf. Accessed 18 Aug. 2018.

269   "LAMICTAL label - FDA." https://www.accessdata.fda.gov/drugsatfda_docs/label/2015/020241s045s051lbl.pdf. Accessed 18 Aug. 2018.

270   "Topamax (topiramate) tablets label - FDA." https://www.accessdata.fda.gov/drugsatfda_docs/label/2012/020844s041lbl.pdf. Accessed 18 Aug. 2018.

271   O'Shaughnessy W B. On the Preparations of the Indian Hemp, or Gunjah - Cannabis Indica Their Effects on the Animal System in Health, and their Utility in the Treatment of Tetanus and other Convulsive Diseases. Prov Med J Retrosp Med Sci. 1843 Feb 4; 5(123): 363–369.

272   Hofmann ME, Frazier CJ. Marijuana, endocannabinoids, and epilepsy: potential and challenges for improved therapeutic intervention. Experimental neurology. 2013;244:43-50. doi:10.1016/j.expneurol.2011.11.047.

273   Perucca E. Cannabinoids in the Treatment of Epilepsy: Hard Evidence at Last? Journal of Epilepsy Research. 2017;7(2):61-76. doi:10.14581/jer.17012.

274   "EPIDIOLEX (cannabidiol) oral solution - FDA." https://www.accessdata.fda.gov/drugsatfda_docs/label/2018/210365lbl.pdf. Accessed 8 Nov. 2018.

275   "FDA-Approved Drug Epidiolex Placed in Schedule V of Controlled ...." 27 Sep. 2018, https://www.justice.gov/opa/pr/fda-approved-drug-epidiolex-placed-schedule-v-controlled-substances-act. Accessed 8 Nov. 2018.

276   Russo EB, Mead AP, Sulak D. Current status and future of cannabis research, in Clinical Researcher. 2015;58–63. 10.14524/CR-15-0004

277   Hall W, Solowij N. Adverse effects of cannabis. Lancet 1998;352:1611-6.

278   Ashton CH. Adverse effects of cannabis and cannabinoids. Br J Anaesth 1999;83:637-49.

279   Handbook of Cannabis Roger Pertwee (ed.) Published in print: 2014 Published Online: January 2015 Publisher: Oxford University Press DOI: 10.1093/

280   Karniol IG, Shirakawa I, Kasinski N, Pfeferman A, Carlini EA. CBD interferes with the effects of delta 9-tetrahydrocannabinol in man. Eur J Pharmacol 1974;28(1):172–7.

281   Lemberger L, Dalton B, Martz R, Rodda B, Forney R. Clinical studies on the interaction of psychopharmacologic agents with marihuana. Ann NY Acad Sci 1976;281: 219–28.

282   The Report of the National Commission on Marihuana and Drug Abuse. Acute Effects of Marihuana. http://druglibrary.net/schaffer/Library/studies/nc/nc1e.htm. Accessed December 6, 2018

283   Volkow ND, Baler RD, Compton WM, Weiss SRB. Adverse Health Effects of Marijuana Use. The New England journal of medicine. 2014;370(23):2219-2227. doi:10.1056/NEJMra1402309.

284   Volkow ND, Baler RD, Compton WM, Weiss SRB. Adverse Health Effects of Marijuana Use. The New England journal of medicine. 2014;370(23):2219-2227. doi:10.1056/NEJMra1402309.

285   Volkow ND, Baler RD, Compton WM, Weiss SRB. Adverse Health Effects

of Marijuana Use. The New England journal of medicine. 2014;370(23):2219-2227. doi:10.1056/NEJMra1402309.

286   Anthony JC,Warner LA,Kessler RC. Comparative epidemiology of dependence on tobacco, alcohol, controlled substances, and inhalants: Basic findings from the National Comorbidity Survey. Experimental and Clinical Psychopharmacology, Vol 2(3), Aug 1994, 244-268

287   De Angelis V, Kockman AC, Weeterings C, Roest M, De Groot PG, Herczenik E, Maas C. Endocannabinoids Control Platelet Activation and Limit Aggregate Formation under Flow. Published: September 29, 2014. https://doi.org/10.1371/journal.pone.0108282

288   Horn JR (PharmD, FCCP), Hansten, PD (PharmD). Drug Interactions with Marijuana. Published December 9, 2014. http://www.pharmacytimes.com/publications/issue/2014/december2014/drug-interactions-with-marijuana   Accessed September 08, 2017

289   Wilens TE, Biederman J, Spencer TJ. Case Study: Adverse Effects of Smoking Marijuana While Receiving Tricyclic Antidepressants. Journal of the American Academy of Child & Adolescent Psychiatry. 1997;36(1):45-48. doi:10.1097/00004583-199701000-00016.

290   Yamreudeewong W, Wong HK, Brausch LM, Pulley KR. Probable Interaction Between Warfarin and Marijuana Smoking. Annals of Pharmacotherapy. 2009;43(7-8):1347-1353. doi:10.1345/aph.1m064.

291   Dr. Edward Group DC, NP, DACBN, DCBCN, DABFM . 5 Health Benefits of Hemp Seed Oil. Last Updated on February 15, 2017. https://www.globalhealingcenter.com/natural-health/5-health-benefits-of-hemp-seed-oil/ Accessed December 6, 2018

292   Susan Patterson. 12 Ways Using Hemp Seed Oil Will Improve Your Health & Your Life. August 16, 2016. http://www.naturallivingideas.com/hemp-seed-oil/. Accessed December 6, 2018

293   http://www.hempfarm.co.nz/health-benefits-of-hemp-seed-oil/ Accessed December 6, 2018

294   http://www.greenremedy.com/sourcing-cbd-marijuana-industrial-hemp-vagaries-federal-law/ Accessed November 20, 2018

295   https://hempmedspx.com/why-full-spectrum-hemp-oil-is-so-important/ Accessed November 20, 2018

296   www.hemp.com/history-of-hemp/ Accessed December 6, 2018

297   Renée Johnson. Hemp as an Agricultural Commodity. Congressional Research Service Report. June 22, 2018. https://fas.org/sgp/crs/misc/RL32725.pdf Accessed December 6 2018

298   Renée Johnson. Hemp as an Agricultural Commodity. Congressional Research Service Report. June 22, 2018. https://fas.org/sgp/crs/misc/RL32725.pdf Accessed December 6 2018

299   http://maui.hawaii.edu/hooulu/2016/01/15/industrial-hemp-a-history-and-

overview-of-the-super-crop-and-its-trillion-dollar-future/ Accessed November 20, 2018

300   https://www.colorado.gov/pacific/agplants/industrial-hemp   Accessed December 6, 2018

301   http://www.kyagr.com/marketing/hemp-pilot.html Accessed December 6, 2018

302   http://maui.hawaii.edu/hooulu/2016/01/15/industrial-hemp-a-history-and-overview-of-the-super-crop-and-its-trillion-dollar-future/ Accessed November 20, 2018

303   Cold, F., Health, E., Disease, H., Disease, L., Management, P. and Conditions, S. (2019). In States With Legal Medical Pot, Teen Use Is Down. [online] WebMD. Available at: https://www.webmd.com/mental-health/addiction/news/20190214/in-states-with-legal-medical-pot-teen-use-is-down#1 [Accessed 27 Apr. 2019].

304   Ksir, C. and Hart, C. (2016). Cannabis and Psychosis: a Critical Overview of the Relationship. Current Psychiatry Reports, 18(2).

305   Inc.com. (2019). Harvard Study Shows Smoking Marijuana Improves Cognitive Function. [online] Available at: https://www.inc.com/cynthia-than/the-surprising-way-to-be-better-at-brain-teasers-a.html [Accessed 27 Apr. 2019].

306   Drugpolicy.org. (2019). [online] Available at: https://www.drugpolicy.org/sites/default/files/DebunkingGatewayMyth_NY_0.pdf [Accessed 27 Apr. 2019].

307   Iowa Now. (2019). UI studies impact of marijuana on driving. [online] Available at: https://now.uiowa.edu/2015/06/ui-studies-impact-marijuana-driving [Accessed 27 Apr. 2019].

308   Reason.org. (2019). [online] Available at: https://reason.org/wp-content/uploads/2018/08/evaluating-research-marijuana-legalization-traffic-accidents.pdf [Accessed 27 Apr. 2019].

309   Aydelotte, J., Brown, L., Luftman, K., Mardock, A., Teixeira, P., Coopwood, B. and Brown, C. (2017). Crash Fatality Rates After Recreational Marijuana Legalization in Washington and Colorado. American Journal of Public Health, 107(8), pp.1329-1331.

310   Ullman, D. (2016). The Effect of Medical Marijuana on Sickness Absence. Health Economics, 26(10), pp.1322-1327.

311   National Academies of Sciences, Engineering, and Medicine. 2017. The Health Effects of Cannabis and Cannabinoids: The Current State of Evidence and Recommendations for Research. Washington, DC: The National Academies Press. https://doi.org/10.17226/24625.

61246261R00098

Made in the USA
Columbia, SC
23 June 2019